Challenges in Pleural Pathology - Diagnostics, Treatment and Research

Edited by Ilze Strumfa, Romans Uljanovs and Boriss Strumfs

Published in London, United Kingdom

Challenges in Pleural Pathology - Diagnostics, Treatment and Research
http://dx.doi.org/10.5772/intechopen.107678
Edited by Ilze Strumfa, Romans Uljanovs and Boriss Strumfs

Contributors
Gilda Diaz-Fuentes, Ivan Alcoholado Boye, Nishant Allena, Pat Arndt, Ralitza Gueorguieva, Richard Kradin, Sindhaghatta Venkatram, Yagnang Kaushikkumar Vyas

First published in London, United Kingdom, 2024 by IntechOpen
IntechOpen is the global imprint of INTECHOPEN LIMITED, registered in England and Wales, registration number: 11086078, 167-169 Great Portland Street, London, W1W 5PF, United Kingdom

British Library Cataloguing-in-Publication Data
A catalogue record for this book is available from the British Library

Additional hard and PDF copies can be obtained from orders@intechopen.com

Challenges in Pleural Pathology - Diagnostics, Treatment and Research
Edited by Ilze Strumfa, Romans Uljanovs and Boriss Strumfs
p. cm.
Print ISBN 978-0-85014-258-7
Online ISBN 978-0-85014-259-4
eBook (PDF) ISBN 978-0-85014-260-0

For EU product safety concerns:
IN TECH d.o.o., Prolaz Marije Krucifikse Kozulić 3, 51000 Rijeka, Croatia,
info@intechopen.com or visit our website at intechopen.com.

Meet the editors

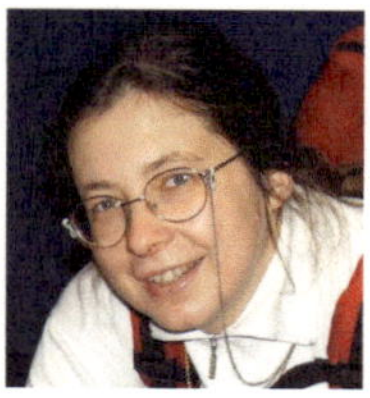

Professor Ilze Strumfa, MD, Ph.D., is an outstanding medical lecturer, actively involved in research in pathology. She graduated from the Medical Academy of Latvia with distinction in 1998, underwent board certification in pathology in 2001, and received a Ph.D. in 2005. Currently, she is a professor and head of the Department of Pathology, Riga Stradins University (RSU), Riga, Latvia. Her 15 years of teaching experience have culminated with the RSU "Lecturer of the Year" Annual Award (2018) and the superior "Teacher of the Year 2023" award of the Latvian Association of Doctors, both given for excellence in university medical teaching. As the head of the Department of Pathology, she is leading a skilled, motivated team of teachers and scientists that have won several awards, including Best Academic Unit (2011), Best Ph.D. Student (2012), and Best Digital Junior Teacher (2016). Prof. Strumfa is an author/co-author of more than 100 peer-reviewed journal articles and 16 chapters in scientific monographs/medical textbooks as well as the editor of 4 monographs. She has participated in several European and national research projects devoted to the development of diagnostic technologies, laboratory training in research, cancer pathology, and tumor microenvironment. Her main research interests include morphological and molecular diagnostics and prognostic assessment of tumors as well as digital pathology and other innovations in pathology and medical education.

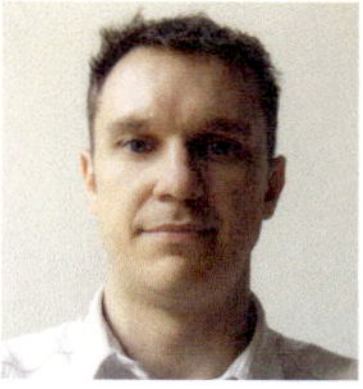

Romans Uljanovs, MD, is a dedicated physician who actively translates his excellent clinical experience into research and medical education, earning the well-deserved respect of colleagues and students. His classes represent attractive, student-centered teaching, simultaneously improving the medical knowledge and logical thinking of attendees. Doctor Uljanovs has developed his scientific experience in two large-scale projects at international and national levels. Notably, he has supervised a team of young teachers to develop gamification as an innovative learning solution in pathology education. Dr. Uljanovs is actively publishing his research in peer-reviewed journals, including *Cells* and the *International Journal of Molecular Pathology.* His main research interests are diagnostic issues and pathogenetic studies, as well as innovations in digital pathology, including game-based approaches in medical teaching.

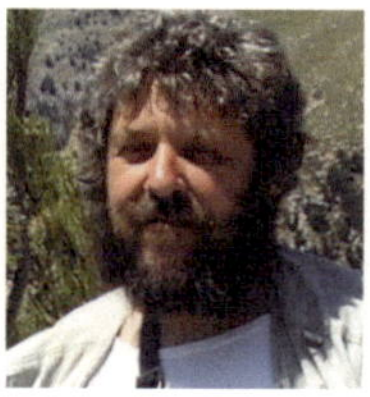

Boriss Strumfs, MSc, Ph.D., is a researcher/leading researcher and lecturer at Latvian Institute of Organic Chemistry and Riga Stradins University (RSU). He graduated with an MSc from the University of Latvia in 1996 and received a Ph.D. in 2012. He has published numerous peer-reviewed scientific articles and five book chapters on pathology (including digital and molecular pathology), issues of organic chemistry, and biochemical events in human disease. B.Strumfs has participated in several national and international research projects in medicine and chemistry and is supervising the research activities of students. His main research interests include biochemical and molecular events in pathology, as well as innovations in organic chemistry.

Contents

Preface

The pleura represents a thin serous membrane that covers the lungs and lines the internal surface of the chest wall, enclosing two pleural cavities. Pleura can be affected by a wide spectrum of pathologies, ranging from effusions, inflammation, and fibrosis to tumors. To reach the correct diagnosis, high awareness of the underlying diseases must be combined with deep knowledge of diagnostic methods, including radiological, biochemical, microbiological, and histological examination. Then, pleural pathology becomes a key to diagnosis.

Considering the clinical importance of pleural pathology, *Challenges in Pleural Pathology – Diagnostics, Treatment and Research* summarizes the classic concepts and innovations in the diagnostics, treatment, and scientific studies of pleural pathology, resulting in a clinically oriented reference as well as a source of ideas for relevant clinical and basic research. It is a collection of review articles grouped into four sections: "Pleural Pathology in Childhood", "Tuberculosis", "Mesothelioma", and "Cutting Edge in Pleural Pathology: New Entities".

In the first section, Chapter 1 presents a review of pleural diseases in newborns and Chapter 2 focuses on the surgical treatment of pleural empyema in children. In newborns, pleural diseases are a rare but significant cause of morbidity and mortality. Congenital chylothorax is the most common type of pleural effusion in neonates. Chapter 1 discusses the diagnostics, differential diagnostics and complex treatment of neonatal chylothorax. Chapter 2 presents useful information on radiological evaluation of pleural empyema in pediatric patients, surgical treatment and postoperative care, as well as postoperative complications and use of fibrinolytic therapy.

Long before *Mycobacterium tuberculosis*, known as Koch's bacillus, was first discovered in 1882 by Robert Koch, tuberculosis was already a major health threat. Evidence of it has been found in 9000-year-old Neolithic human remains. Tuberculosis has been identified in Egyptian mummies, sparing not even pharaohs. It is said that pharaoh Akhenaten and his wife Nefertiti both died from tuberculosis around 1330 BC. Nowadays, tuberculosis is considered a curable disease, and health care benefits from outstanding diagnostic possibilities. Nevertheless, according to World Health Organization (WHO) data, 1.3 million people died from tuberculosis in 2022, ranking it as the second leading infectious killer worldwide after COVID-19. The global estimates of tuberculosis cases in 2022 reached 10.6 million. Tuberculosis is not a solved problem even in Europe. In 2021, tuberculosis mortality in the WHO European region increased compared to 2020, and the declining incidence curve has stalled for the first time in 20 years. Thus, the numbers of new and relapsed tuberculosis cases in the WHO European Region were 216,368 in 2019, 164,187 cases in 2020, and 166,000 in 2021. Considering the persisting clinical importance of tuberculosis, Chapter 3 targets pleural tuberculosis, the second most common form of extrapulmonary tuberculosis. The analysis of pathogenetic mechanisms is followed by an insight into clinical manifestations of pleural tuberculosis and a well-illustrated description of radiological findings via chest X-ray, pleural ultrasonography, and computed tomography. The chapter also details the laboratory assessment of pleural fluid and pleural biopsy and describes combined anti-tuberculous, anti-inflammatory, and surgical treatment.

The most frequent primary malignant pleural neoplasm is malignant mesothelioma, arising from mesothelial cells that line the pleura. Mesothelioma is known for its strong epidemiological association with asbestos exposure, peculiar encasing gross growth pattern, difficult surgical treatment, and dismal prognosis. Considering the limited treatment efficacy, mesothelioma represents an unmet need for the healthcare system. However, recent years have yielded significant discoveries, e.g., on germline mutations in *BAP1* gene coding BRCA1-associated protein 1, pathogenetic role of inflammation, and innovative treatment approaches (e.g., immune checkpoint blockers and PARP inhibitors). Chapter 4 examines the general characteristics of pleural mesothelioma, which represents more than 80% of all mesothelioma cases. This chapter provides an insight into the epidemiology and pathogenesis of pleural mesothelioma, followed by a description of clinical presentation, imaging modalities, biomarkers, and invasive diagnostic modalities. Surgical and systemic treatment are characterized as well. The clinical point of view is further complemented by research trends in Chapter 5, which highlights the association between talc exposure and mesothelioma, expanding the classic scope of mesothelioma risk factors, dominated by asbestos.

Medicine is a dynamic, constantly developing field. Each new discovery brings benefits but encounters new problems. Lung transplantation and transplantation of hematopoietic stem cells are outstanding medical achievements. However, transplant recipients can develop unusual, delayed, chronic, non-infectious complications. Chapter 6 provides a comprehensive review of post-transplantation complications in pleura, namely, serositis and pleuroparenchymal fibroelastosis. In the given context, serositis represents a pleural effusion that cannot be attributed to infection, cardiac dysfunction, volume overload, or neoplasm. Pleuroparenchymal fibroelastosis mainly affects the upper lobes as fibrous thickening of pleura and bands of fibrous tissue extending from the pleura to the hilum, contracting the affected lobes. Both these entities are characterized by delayed onset, incompletely understood pathogenesis, a hypothetic component of graft-versus-host disease, and lack of effective treatment. Higher awareness of serositis and pleuroparenchymal fibroelastosis is mandatory to prompt diagnostics and research.

The book has been created by a truly global team of doctors and scientists from Bulgaria, Chile, India, as well as several universities and clinics from the United States, including Harvard Medical School, University of Minnesota, and BronxCare Health System of New York. We would like to sincerely thank all the authors for their excellent contributions, clinical experience, and sharp minds.

Last but not least, we express our sincere gratitude to the IntechOpen editorial team for their continuous support and professional help throughout all stages of book production.

"Everything should be made as simple as possible, but not simpler".

Albert Einstein

Ilze Strumfa, MD, Ph.D.
Professor,
Department of Pathology,
Riga Stradins University,
Riga, Latvia

Romans Uljanovs, MD
Department of Pathology,
Riga Stradins University,
Riga, Latvia

Boriss Strumfs, MSc, Ph.D.
Latvian Institute of Organic Synthesis,
Department of Pathology,
Riga Stradins University,
Riga, Latvia

Section 1

Pleural Pathology in Childhood

Chapter 1

Pleural Diseases in Newborn Infants

Ralitza Gueorguieva

Abstract

Pleural diseases are rare in the neonatal period, but sometimes are associated with significant morbidity and mortality. Congenital chylothorax is the most common type of pleural effusion in neonates. The diagnostic approach to neonatal chylothorax and neonatal pleural effusions are discussed in detail. The management of congenital chylothorax is challenging, because it includes prenatal procedures, diet, drug treatment, and surgery. Summarized treatment protocol gives information about the most important therapeutic measures, according to the postnatal age and clinical evolution. Brief description of the other types of pleural effusions is provided.

Keywords: neonate, pleura, effusion, chylothorax, congenital

1. Introduction

Pleural diseases in the neonatal period are rare, but some of them are associated with significant morbidity and mortality. The most common neonatal pleural disease is the chylothorax – congenital and acquired. There is lack of uniform guidelines for the prenatal and postnatal treatment of this condition. The aim of this chapter is to summarize the clinical experience, provide up to date knowledge, and delineate future perspectives.

1.1 Neonatal pleural effusions

Pleural effusion is defined as fluid accumulation in the pleural space between the parietal and visceral pleura. There are many conditions in the neonatal period associated with changes of the pulmonary venous hydrostatic pressure, lymphatic pressure, blood oncotic pressure, and local tissue trauma or inflammation all of them leading to the development of pleural effusion [1]. The incidence of pleural effusions in neonates varies between 5.5/10000 to 2.2% in different clinical settings [2, 3]. The prevalence of pleural effusion is high in neonates admitted to the NICU (neonatal intensive care unit) [2].

1.2 Classification of neonatal pleural effusions

About 10–30% of neonatal pleural effusions are identified prenatally, and up to 90% are postnatally acquired [4, 5].

1.3 Prenatally acquired pleural effusions

The most common types and causes of congenital pleural effusion are as follows [6]:

- Immune and nonimmune hydrops – abnormal fetal liquid collection in a minimum of two anatomic locations. Fetal hydrops could be immune-mediated (Rh incompatibility) or nonimmune (genetic syndromes, metabolic diseases, hematologic disorders (alpha thalassemia), and infections).

- Chromosomal diseases – most commonly Turner and Down syndrome. Turner syndrome is a condition, when one of the X chromosomes is missing or partially missing, and in Down syndrome, there is an extra copy of chromosome 21.

- Congenital pneumonia.

- Congenital chylothorax.

- Congenital heart failure.

- Congenital nonchylous-isolated pleural effusion.

- Infections – cytomegalovirus, herpes simplex virus, toxoplasmosis, and coxsackie viruses.

- Pulmonary malformations – bronchopulmonary sequestration, pulmonary lymphangiectasia, pulmonary lymphatic hypoplasia, and congenital pulmonary airway malformation [7, 8].

- Rare causes – obstructive uropathy [9, 10], congenital malignancies [11], thoracic hamartoma [12, 13], and intrapericardial teratomas [14].

The incidence of congenital isolated pleural effusion is about 1:12,000 to 1:15,000 [15]. Isolated nonchylous effusions without concomitant pathologic conditions are very rare [16]. The most common type of congenital isolated pleural effusion is the congenital chylous pleural effusion [17].

1.4 Postnatally acquired pleural effusions

- Severe sepsis – pleural effusion could be associated very rare with severe neonatal sepsis [18].

- COVID-19-related neonatal pleural effusion [19].

- Parapneumonic effusions and empyema – positive pleural culture or purulent effusion with elevated white blood cells (WBC) and higher percentage of polymorphonuclears (PMN), high protein content, and presence of bacteria. Pleural effusions are mostly seen in sepsis and pneumonia, caused by *Staphylococcus aureus*, *Streptococcus pneumoniae*, *Streptococcus pyogenes*, *Bacteroides fragilis*, *Acinetobacter* spp., *Enterobacter aerogenes*, *Escherichia coli*, *Klebsiella* spp.,

Pseudomonas aeruginosa, and *Acinetobacter caloasceticus* [20]. The development of neonatal empyema goes through three stages – exudative, fibrinopurulent, and organizational. Chest ultrasound is extremely helpful in the diagnosis and follow-up of parapneumonic effusion [21].

- Hemothorax – presence of blood in the pleural space.

- Congestive heart failure could be complicated by bilateral pleural effusions with characteristics of a transudate – total protein content of the fluid <30 g/l and WBC <2000/mm^3.

- Acquired chylothorax – the most common cause is cardiothoracic surgery with an incidence of 2–3% [22], diaphragmatic hernia, and perinatal trauma due to stretching of the chest wall during resuscitation. In traumatic injury, the latent period for chyle accumulation could be 2–10 days [3, 23, 24]. The reported incidence of chylothorax after cardio-thoracic surgery in children is reported to be between 0.85 and 6.6% [25, 26]. This pathophysiological mechanism causes injury to the thoracic duct [4, 5, 27, 28].

- PICC (percutaneously inserted central venous line) extravasation – the analysis of pleural fluid usually shows an increased content of glucose and triglycerides, depending on the composition of infusion solutions and low cell count. Percutaneously inserted central venous lines are widely used in all neonatal departments for prolonged venous infusion, use of vasoactive drugs (catecholamines), and parenteral nutrition. The placement is easy, but some common complications could happen such as catheter-associated infection, pericardial effusion, pleural effusion, ascites, venous thrombosis, and phlebitis [29, 30]. Some of the complications could be avoided by precise placement of the catheter. The tip should be in the superior vena cava or inferior vena cava and not advancing to the right atrium. When the catheter is used for prolonged time, regular X-ray controls should be done, because spontaneous migration of catheter is also possible. The prevalence of parenteral fluid extravasation from central venous line was reported to be 0.05–1% [31]. The most common mechanisms are perforation of blood vessels during the placement procedure, retrograde passage of a central venous catheter into the lymphatic duct, erosion of veins especially in cases of spontaneous catheter migration, and, in extremely premature infants, hyperosmotic endothelial damage, leading to increased vascular permeability [32–34].

- UVC (umbilical venous catheter) extravasation.

2. Diagnosis of neonatal pleural effusion

The diagnosis of pleural effusion is based on the following:

- Antenatal presentation – ultrasonography is very useful for the diagnosis of hydrops fetus, congenital heart diseases, pulmonary abnormalities, and fetal pleural effusions. Long standing effusions developed prior to the 20th gestational week may result in pulmonary hypoplasia.

- Clinical symptoms – respiratory distress syndrome, worsening respiratory failure, hypoxemia, diminished breathing sounds unilateral or bilateral, and dullness to percussion. Small effusions could be asymptomatic, and the pleural effusion could be incidentally diagnosed.

- X-ray and ultrasound findings typical for pleural effusion – the thoracic X-rays of the newborn infants usually are made in the supine position, so the pleural effusions usually are visualized as a diffuse homogenous density over the whole lung. These findings can be very easily confirmed using an ultrasound examination, which could be provided bedside and is also very useful for follow-up of the amount of pleural fluid and, respectively, the therapeutic results, without repositioning the infant [35].

- Analysis of pleural effusion fluid – appearance, pH, density, presence of red blood cells (RBC), WBC, protein content, glucose, lactate dehydrogenase (LDH), and triglycerides. Pleural effusion could be chylous and nonchylous. The nonchylous effusion could be exudate or transudate. Transudate is produced due to imbalances in hydrostatic and oncotic pressure, in neonates frequently is seen in venous hypertension or obstruction due to congenital heart disease, in pulmonary malformations, hypoalbuminemia, extravasation from venous lines.

Differential diagnosis is based mainly on the pleural fluid characteristics:

- Transudate – total protein: <30 g/l, WBC: <2000/mm^3, predominance of mononuclear cells.

- Exudative fluid – high protein content, predominance of PMN, pathogens visible on Gram's stain.

- Chylothorax (criteria, defined by Buttiker et al. [23, 36, 37]).

  1. Total white cell count: > 1000 cells/μl.

  2. Lymphocyte fraction: > 80%.

  3. Triglyceride levels: > 110 mg/dl (1.24 mmol/l).

Milky pleural fluid could be seen in the following cases [38]:

- Chylothorax.

- Empyema.

- Leakage from the central venous line.

- Milk leakage from perforated esophagus.

- Trauma to the thoracic duct – after surgical interventions or following traumatic vaginal delivery in breech presentation.

3. Congenital chylothorax

3.1 Incidence

The incidence of congenital chylothorax is reported to be 1:5775 to 1:100,000 live births, 1:10,000–1:24,000, 1:7300–1:10,000, 4 per 100,000 live births [39]. This is the most common form of pleural effusion in the perinatal period [39–42]. The chylothorax is defined as accumulation of chyle in the in the pleural cavity [43]. H. Linner and Stewart are the first authors who described a congenital chylothorax in newborn [44]. In 1928, the first prenatal diagnosis of congenital chylothorax was reported [45]. Congenital chylothorax could be presented prenatally by the development of hydrops fetalis in one-third of the cases and has mainly bilateral pleural involvement. The pathophysiology is based on different abnormalities of the lymphatic system – maldevelopment or obstruction [1, 3, 27, 43, 46–48]. It can be idiopathic or may be associated with different genetic diseases [49]. Anomalies and malformations can be identified in 80% of the cases [40, 42, 50–54]. In a systematic review of 753 cases with congenital chylothorax, chromosomal diseases were identified in 18% and associated anomalies in 29% [55]. In a clinical cohort of 62 neonates with chylothorax, congenital pleural effusions were congenital in 32 and 68% acquired. Secondary etiologies were more frequent than congenital [3]. In another clinical setting, chylothorax was the most common cause of neonatal pleural effusion (9/21, 43%), 44% in congenital and 56% in acquired. The range of occurrence age was 5–46 days for congenital chylothorax and 2–44 days for acquired [4].

3.2 Causes of congenital chylothorax

- Idiopathic [56]
- Congenital malformations of lymphatics.
    - Lymphangiomatosis.
    - Lymhangiectasia.
    - Atresia of thoracic duct.
    - Cystic hygroma.
- Associated with syndromes.
    - Down syndrome.
    - Noonan syndrome.

Autosomal dominant inherited disorder presented with abnormal facial features, congenital heart disease and growth issues, developmental delay, muscle and bone abnormalities, and lymphedema.

Turner syndrome.

Gorham-Stout syndrome [57].

Vanishing bone disease, a rare disorder of unknown etiology, presented by destruction of the osseous matrix and proliferation of vascular structures, resulting in destruction and absorption of bones.

Yellow nail syndrome.

Very rare condition defined by the presence of slow growing, yellow and dystrophic nails, lymphedema, and respiratory diseases, which may be a genetic disorder.

Other syndromes.

X-linked myotubular myopathy [52].

Missense mutation in integrin alpha and beta [58, 59].

In meta-analysis published in 2022, 217 (29%) of the cases were with associated congenital anomalies and 51% of them are of pulmonary and lymphatic origin – congenital pulmonary lymhangiectasia (20%), pulmonary hypoplasia (20%), and extrapulmonary lymphatic dysplasia (7%). Congenital heart diseases and malformations of the arteriovenous system were diagnosed in 52 cases (24%).Chromosomal aberrations were found in 118/753 cases (18%), the most common were Down, Turner, and Noonan syndromes [55]. Different anomalies of the lymphatic system could be responsible for the development of chylothorax [60–62].

3.3 Pathophysiology of congenital chylothorax

The human lymphatic system is involved in the transport of lipids to the systemic circulation and return of excess fluid, lymphocytes, and proteins from the interstitial spaces to the circulation [37, 62]. The name of the lymphatic body fluid – chyle – originates from the Greek word for juice (Chylus). It has milky appearance, undergoes alkaline reaction, and has bacteriostatic properties. Chyle contains mainly fat (phospholipids, cholesterol, and long-chain triglycerides in the form of chylomicrones), electrolytes, proteins, immunoglobulins, glucose, and lymphocytes. The protein content is over 3 g/l, and the electrolyte composition is similar to that of serum [42]. The cell count is >1000 cells/μL, and the lymphocyte count varies from 400 to 6800 mm^3, mainly T lymphocytes [63, 64]. The main source of chyle are digested fatty foods in the small intestine. Dietary fats are absorbed by the intestinal enterocytes in the form of chylomicrons and transported by the lymph vessels. Lymph vessels from the lower part of the body confluence and form the thoracic duct, which is placed on the right side of the vertebral column (chylothorax is more commonly seen on the right side) [37]. Flow through the thoracic duct is highly variable, depending on the enteral feeding (14 ml/h in the fasting period and up to 100 ml/h in postprandial state) [65]. Thoracic duct flow is sensible to splanchnic and vagal stimulation. Serotonin, norepinephrine, histamine, dopamine, and acetylcholine all increase the duct contraction and chyle flow [66]. The thoracic duct transports a large volume of chyle daily, and if the flow is compromised by different reasons, a rapid accumulation of chyle could occur [65]. In case of malfunction or obstruction of the lymphatic system, the chyle accumulates and bursts through the pleura [37]. The long persisting chylothorax is associated with significant chronic loss of lymphocytes and immunoglobulins and, respectively, immunodeficiency as well as malnutrition due to loss of fats and fat-soluble vitamins. Severe hypoimmunoglobulinemia could develop [67–69]. After 14 days of chylous drainage, lymphocyte depletion was observed. In a large series of 178 infants, low lymphocyte count was associated with culture positive sepsis [5]. Chylothorax-associated infections are rare due to the bacteriostatic properties of the chyle [36]. The most serious consequences of fetal chylothorax are pulmonary hypoplasia, congestive heart failure, and hydrops [70, 71]. Hydrops effusion fetalis is presented by significant fluid accumulation in the fetus and other specific antenatal ultrasound findings, such as skin edema, pericardial and pleural effusions, ascites, and polyhydramnios. In a patient setting of 598 infants with hydrops, the cause was identified as congenital chylothorax in 3.2%; other causes were congenital cardiac malformations and heart rate abnormalities, twin-twin transfusion syndrome, anomalies, chromosomal diseases, transplacental viral infections, and fetal anemia [72]. Congenital chylothorax can cause nonimmune hydrops from a combination of increased capillary filtration rate and reduced lymphatic clearance due to disturbed vena cava blood flow or following the mass effect of the chylous effusion, which leads to compromised cardiac function [73, 74]. Hypoalbuminemia, following the loss of albumin with chyle into the pleural space, could decrease the capillary osmotic pressure and leads to the development of fetal hydrops [74]. Lymphangiectasia and other congenital lymphatic disorders can also present usually as bilateral chylothorax as a result of obstruction to the lymphatic flow. Cystic hygromas cause mass compression effect and impairment of the lymphatic drainage and venous return to the heart [75].

3.4 Clinical presentation of congenital chylothorax

1. Congenital chylothorax usually is diagnosed in the antenatal period as a space occupying lesion, with 50%, presenting with pleural effusion on day 1 of life [23,24]. Prenatally existing effusions could lead to pulmonary hypoplasia, and the increased intrathoracic pressure interferes with the swallowing and development of polyhydramnios [76]. One recently published meta-analysis included 753 cases from 157 publications. About 71% of the included infants were born preterm, intrauterine death occurred in 42 cases, and termination of pregnancy was reported in 13 cases. The median age of prenatal diagnosis was 28.8 (16–38) weeks, and the median age of prenatal interventions was 29.7 weeks (17–38) [56].

2. Postnatal clinical presentation is respiratory distress syndrome and mild to severe hypoxemia [77]. Clinical manifestation depends on the rate of chyle leakage and the duration of chylothorax. Rapid accumulation of fluid in the pleural cavity results in significantly increased positive pleural pressure and cardiorespiratory distress [38]. In the postnatal period, chylothorax impairs ventilation and oxygenation, and cardiac failure could occur due to increased venous pressure. Hypoalbuminemia and nutritional depletion are the consequences of prolonged pleural drainage and chronic loss of protein and fat. The risk of infections is increased due to the loss of lymphocytes and immunoglobulins.

3.5 Diagnosis of chylothorax

1. Ultrasound diagnosis of fetal pleural effusion and associated conditions such as polyhydramnios or hydrops in the most severe cases.

2. X-ray and ultrasound diagnosis of pleural effusion in the postnatal period.

3. Complex analysis of pleural fluid.

The diagnosis of chylothorax based on the analysis of pleural fluid is made according to the criteria, defined by Buttiker et al. – triglycerides above 110 mg/dl (1.24 mmol/l) and elevated cell number (> 1000 cells/µl on the fluid microscopy and > 80% lymphocytes) [23]. The amount of triglycerides in the pleural fluid reflects the presence of chylomicrons, but depends strongly on the oral milk and fat intake which is the reason for diagnostic difficulties in some patients, especially premature infants. The lipoprotein electrophoresis is the golden standard for diagnosis when the other data are inconclusive (triglyceride levels in the range 0.56–1.24 mmol/l). The chylomicrons are identified on the base of their charge and mass under electrical field, and they are uncharged and remain at their original place [78]. Pleural fluid triglyceride levels <0.56 mmol/l exclude chylothorax [79]. In about 14% of congenital chylothoraces, it is possible to find a low level of triglycerides (< 1,24 mmol/l), when the age of the baby is very small and if the enteral nutrition is totally absent or is in very small amounts [80]). When the results from the pleural fluid are inconclusive, a relation pleural fluid/serum could be used: fluid/serum triglycerides>1, fluid/serum cholesterol <1, and fluid triglycerides to cholesterol ratio > 1 [23, 36, 37]. Chyle separates in three layers in standing position: chylomicrons form the upper creamy layer, the medium layer is milky, and the bottom layer contains cellular elements, predominantly lymphocytes [64]. In empyema, a clear supernatant is formed after centrifugation [49, 63, 81]. Pseudochylothorax should be included in the differential diagnosis – when long persistence of pleural effusion and cholesterol crystals are formed, but the thoracic duct is fully intact. When this is the case, the fluid could be cleared out by adding 1–2 ml of ethyl ether [78].

4. Management of neonatal pleural effusions

Pleural effusions following central venous line extravasation are treated with removal of the central venous line and chest drainage if there is a clinical indication. The resolution happens in few days. In empyema cases, the treatment consists of chest drain, eventually urokinase fibrinolysis, thoracotomy, or video-assisted thoracoscopy, especially when the treatment with chest drainage and or without fibrinolysis has failed [21].

4.1 Prenatal management of congenital chylothorax

- Ultrasound diagnosis of prenatal pleural effusion.
- Diagnosis of hydrops, associated anomalies, and chromosomal diseases.
- Decision making about palliative or active treatment depending on the associated clinical conditions.
- The active treatment requires placing of prenatal thoraco-amniotic shunting with pigtail catheter in an experienced center or fetal pleurodesis with OK-432.
- Diet modification for the mother.

4.1.1 Prenatal treatment procedures

Infants with ultrasound diagnosis of chylothorax before 34th week of gestation who received prenatal therapy have better postnatal adaptation and improved postnatal outcomes [82]. Therapeutic measures in the prenatal period include maternal dietary modification [83], repeated thoracocentesis [70, 84, 85], thoraco-amniotic shunting [86], and pleurodesis with OK-432 [87–90]. The results of prenatal treatment depends on the time of diagnosis, effusion volume, presence of hydrops, and high-grade lung compression. The risk of development of pulmonary hypoplasia is highest before 24th week of gestation. If the effusion is small and develops in more advanced pregnancy, expectant management is recommended [85]. Thoraco-amniotic shunting was first described by Rodeck et al. as a method to decompress the fetal lungs [91], allowing better lung development. The survival following pleuroamniotic shunting has been reported to be between 47 and 70% [92–97]. Resolution of hydrops following intervention was associated with improved survival. Displacement of the shunt occurred in 23% of the cases [98]. Antenatal treatment was performed in 316/512 (62%) prenatally diagnosed cases, 40% pleural punctuations, 43% thoraco-amniotic shunting, and 5% both procedures [55]. Pleural punctuations prior to delivery could prevent perinatal asphyxia. Picone et al. described 44 intrauterine shunted patients with recurrent punctuations until birth [86]. Chen et al. published 17 cases with intrauterine pleural punctuations; some of them performed immediately before birth and these patients showed better postpartum adaptation [99]. A total of 87 cases were treated with fetal intrapleural instillation of OK-432. OK-432 (Picibanil) is a lyophilized preparation of a low-virulence human-derived strain of group A *Streptococcus pyogenes*, used as a sclerosing agent. There are a lot of reports, demonstrating good results of this fetal intervention [87–90, 100]. Tanemura et al. first published this method in 2001 [88], and Yang et al. [101] reported the results from the treatment of 45 fetuses – 31 fetuses survived the procedure and showed complete (eight cases) and partial (23 cases) response and were followed up until the delivery, 16 (51.6%) survived more than 1 month, and 15(48%) died before reaching the age of 1 month. Lee et al. [82] reported about using three different modalities for prenatal treatment – pleurodesis, thoracocentesis, and thoraco-amniotic shunting. Treatment with instillation of maternal blood into the fetal pleural cavity has been reported [102].

4.2 Postnatal course of the disease and postnatal management

- If it is possible, delivery should happen in a facility with III Level NICU.
- Management in the delivery room.
- If the respiratory insufficiency immediately after delivery is severe, needle aspiration of the pleural fluid should be done in delivery room, followed by thoracocentesis and continuous drainage.
- Initial postnatal treatment: [56]
- Asymptomatic infants with small effusions should be placed on close clinical observation.
- Symptomatic infants should receive different basic therapeutic measures, depending on the clinical condition:
    - Oxygen therapy.
    - CPAP (continuous positive airway pressure) using facial mask or nasal prongs.

- Noninvasive ventilation.
- Intubation and mechanical ventilation.
- Empiric antibiotic therapy.
- Infants with nonchylous pleural effusion and significant fluid losses (greater than 6 ml/kg/hour) through the thorax drainage should receive fluid replacement with normal saline and appropriate amount of potassium. Volume loss should be calculated every 8 to 12 hours.

4.2.1 Treatment of chylothorax

- Draining the chylothorax.
- Needle aspirations.
- Tube thoracostomy – chest tubes 10–12 fr, pigtail catheters 8.5 fr or greater. The chest tube should be inserted in the midaxillary line, 5th and 6th intercostal space, directed posteriorly and connected to low pressure suction device.
- Continuous suction drainage could cause volume depletion, loss of electrolytes, proteins, albumin, immunoglobulins, and lymphocytes. After prolonged pleural drainage in chylous effusion, significant losses of fluid, electrolytes, proteins, immunoglobulins, and lymphocytes occur [103]. Meta-analysis including large number of patients reported that pleural punctions (drainages) were performed in 64% (438/681) of the cases, and the indication was hypoxemia and increased work of breathing. The mean duration of pleural drainages, documented in 225 newborns, was on average 20 days (range 1–150) [55].
    - Adequate ventilation.
    - Total parenteral nutrition – in the initial stage of treatment and after unsuccessful MCT (medium-chain triglycerides) formula diet.
    - Fluid therapy adjusted to the thorax drainage losses.
    - Albumin replacement – level should be checked once per week.
    - Replacement of coagulation factors – levels should be checked once per week.
    - Immunglobulin replacement – the target level of IgG should be 500 mg/dl, initial dosing – 400–600 mg/kg.
    - Diet measures Diet measures – enteral feeding with MCT (medium-chain triglycerides) formulas: this type of dietary approach could reduce the chyle flow and chylous effusions. MCT are directly absorbed in the portal vein system, bypassing the lymphatic system and reducing the volume and lipid content of the pleural fluid [46]. If the drainage of chyle continues more than a week on MCT formula, feeding trial of total parenteral nutrition should be done.

MCT formulas have shown to be effective in decreasing the chyle flow and resolutions of chylous effusions [25, 104, 105]. Low fat formulas or fat-free human milk, produced with centrifugation and supplementation with median chain triglycerides, could also be used [106]. MCT formulas or total parenteral nutrition can resolve 50% of the cases [23]. Analysis of a large clinical cohort showed that mechanical ventilation was needed in 56% (381/681) and total parenteral nutrition in 44% (296/681), with mean 21 days (range 2–81). MCT diet was given in 315 cases (46%) and was initiated at the mean age of 21 days (range 7–68) and was done for mean 37 days (range 5–50 days). In 96 cases, a prenatal MCT diet of the mother was reported [55].

4.2.1.1 Medications

Octreotide is used in infants failing to respond after 1 to 2 weeks of dietary treatment. Octreotide is a synthetic somatostatin analogue, reducing the intestinal blood flow and chyle production. Use of octreotide for the management of congenital chylothorax was first reported by Young et al. from Canada [107]. In neonates, octreotide is used for the treatment of persisitent neonatal hyperinsulinism [108]. The mechanism of action is reduction in gastric, pancreatic, and intestinal secretions as well as intestinal absorption [109]. Cochrane review summarized the published data on the use of octreotide and concluded that many clinical trials generally demonstrated resolution of chylothorax after octreotide treatment. Time of initiation, dose, duration, and frequency of doses showed significant variations – subcutaneously at 10–70 μg/kg/day given in 6–24 hourly doses or as continuous intravenous infusion between 0.3 and 10 μg/kg/hour. The duration of treatment varies between 4 and 21 days and is mostly guided by clinical response [110]. Octreotide is associated with adverse effects such as arrhythmias, hyperglycemia, transient hypothyroididsm, and impairement of liver function, necrotizing enterocolitis [111], hypoxemia, and pulmonary hypertension [112]. Octreotide continues to be used as off-label medication in the management of congenital chylothorax. The initial dose of octreotide is 1 μcg/kg/h and should be increased, depending on the response by 1 μg/kg/h until a response is verified or until the dose reaches 10 μg/kg/h. The response is classified as positive if there is at least 25% reduction in output. In a case of positive response, the infusion should continue with the same rate for 7–10 days, followed by slow tampering over 1 week. If the maximal dose is not effective for 2–3 days, it should be tapered off. After closing the drainage and removing the chest tubes, enteral feeding with human milk should begin after 1 week at least [103].The treatment of chylothorax with somatostatin and octreotide (somatostatin analogue) was suggested for the first time by Goto et al. in 2003 [113]. Cleveland et al. reported a series of 13 infants treated with both drugs (somatostatin and octreotide) [114]. After that, a lot of data about somatostatin and octreotide treatment were accumulated. The mean duration of octreotide treatment in 138 infants was 22 days (range 3–151 in 76 patients), and the mean age at the start of the therapy was between 2 and 109 days. These medications could be applied intravenously or subcutaneously. The initial intravenous dosage should be 3–4 μg/kg/h, and the maximum dosage 6–12 μg/kg/h. The initial dose of subcutaneous injection could be between 1 and 40 μg/kg/day and the maximal dose 24–70 μg/kg/24 h [55]. In a cohort reported by Cannizarro et al., three newborns were treated with somatostatin, and the start dose was 3.5 μg/kg/h and was gradually increased to 12 μg/kg/h [115]. The medication could be given subcutaneously at the same dose at 6- to 8-hour intervals. Adverse effects of octreotide have been reported in 14% of infants with chylothorax [116]. Octreotide reduces the insulin release, so close monitoring of blood glucose is needed. A systematic review of 753 patients with congenital chylothorax reported that, of the 138 infants, treated with octreotide, 78% had resolution of chylothorax without the need for surgical intervention [55]. In a large case series of 178 infants with chylous effusions, 172 were treated with thorax drainage and nutritional measures, and six infants were not treated. About 45 infants were treated with octreotide, and 21 patients underwent surgery. There was no additional benefit of octreotide over dietary measures [5]. Another systematic review reported that octreotide is safe and effective intervention, showing decrease or cessation of chylous drainage in 50% of the cases [117].

Sildenafil (phosphodiesterase 5 blocker) could be effective for the treatment of pulmonary hypertension and has the potential to enhance the lymphatic vessel growth and/or remodeling, resolving the lymphatic obstruction and chylothorax [56];

Sirolimus (rapamycin) – this is a macrolide compound, inhibiting (mTOR) kinase. It is used to treat vascular malformations and has the potential to slow the growth of abnormal lymphatic vessels. Effective treatment of chylothoraces in older children and adults was described, but the dosing information for neonates and infants is very limited. In a recent study, age-appropriate dosing regimens for neonates and infants were identified [118].

Propanolol (beta blocker) [119–121] – evidence is still insufficient to recommend routine use in newborn infants.

4.2.1.2 Surgical interventions

- Redirection of chyle – pleuroperitoneal shunt and diaphragmatic fenestration.

- Obstruction of chyle flow into the chest (thoracic duct ligation or embolization) – after lymphoangiography and locating of the rupture site of ductus thoracicus, a definitive surgical management could be performed – direct ligation of the thoracic duct [23, 24, 78].

- Pleurodesis – a procedure to obliterate the pleural space. The pleural cavity should be drained, and after that, a chemical substance is instilled causing inflammation and fibrosis. The following agents have been used in infants: iodopovidone, fibrin glue, *Streptococcus pyogenes* A3 (OK-432), tetracycline derivatives (oxytetracycline doxycycline), talc, and other agents [122–129]. Fetal drainage plus subsequent pleurodesis with OK-432 was shown as a promising approach with 67% survival [55].

4.2.2 Summary about the management of chylothorax in newborn infants

4.2.2.1 Prenatal intervention

- Ultrasound diagnosis of pleural effusion/hydrops fetalis [55].

- Diagnosis of chromosomal diseases/malformations.

- Decision about active or palliative treatment.

- Consider prenatal thoraco-amniotic shunting or pleural punctuations.
- Consider pleurodesis (OK-432).

4.2.2.2 Birth

- Active treatment or palliative care.
- Respiratory support.
- Pleural drainage.

4.2.2.3 Diagnosis of congenital chylothorax

- Lymphocytes >80%.
- High level of triglyceride.
- Document fluid losses to estimate fluid balance and electrolyte, protein, and immunoglobulin losses.

4.2.2.4 Weeks 1–4

- Treatment strategies in confirmed cases.
- Start with total parenteral nutrition.
- Removing the pigtail catheter placed antenatal or placement of new pleural drainage.
- Initiate MCT diet very slowly, depending on pleural fluid and maintain the drainages.
- If pleural fluid increases, go back to total parenteral nutrition.

4.2.2.5 Weeks 5 and 6

- MCT diet until full enteral nutrition.
- If not possible, begin octreotide treatment intravenously or subcutaneously.
- If not successful, consider surgical treatment: pleurodesis or surgical ligation of the thoracic duct or both.
- Antibiotics for prophylaxis/treatment.
- Immunoglobulins every 2–4 weeks to maintain the physiological levels.

4.2.2.6 Practice points

- Prenatal interventions in experienced perinatal centers could improve survival in severe fetal chylothorax.
- The therapeutic approach should be stepwise, depending on chylothorax severity and treatment risks.

4.2.2.7 Prognosis of congenital chylothorax

The neonatal chylothorax is associated with high mortality rate (20–60% and 30–70%), especially when associated with other comorbidities [42, 56, 130]. The highest mortality rate was observed in patients with hydrops fetalis, severe congenital conditions, and serious lymphatic abnormalities. Risk factors for death in acquired chylothorax are prematurity and infection [42]. In 462 cases (68%), the resolution of the chylothorax was complete, and in 34/44 cases following intrauterine intervention, time of complete regression was at mean 28 days (1–148). In those treated prenatally, resolving of the pleural effusion was noted around 24 weeks of gestation (19–26) [55].

4.2.2.8 Follow-up

About 133 neonates with chylothorax were followed up for 1–144, mean 14.7 months. The longest clinical observation included six cases followed up to the age of 12 [131]. Recurrence of pleural effusions was not reported. Long-term observations revealed two cases with later development of interstitial infiltrations, one – bronchial asthma, one – pulmonary obstructive disease, and one with pleural fibrosis.

5. Discussion

Neonatal pleural pathology is relatively rare, but some of the clinical cases impose significant diagnostic and therapeutic challenges. The most common type of neonatal pleural effusion is chylothorax. Important clinical issue is the fact that the majority of infants with congenital chylothorax have a significant comorbidity, presented by chromosomal diseases and malformations. This requires more complex clinical approach including the efforts of obstetricians, neonatologists, pediatric surgeons, and clinical genetics specialists. Precise diagnosis of accompanying conditions is very important, regarding the indications for prenatal interventions and the extent of postnatal management. The treatment of nonchylous effusions is easier, but the therapeutic protocol especially for congenital chylothorax is more complicated. There is a general agreement in the literature and clinical practice in different clinical settings about the necessity of a prenatal procedures in some cases, stepwise postnatal approach with a clear priority of pleural drainage and dietary measures. Medical treatment should include preferably drugs with a greater experience of use in the neonatal period, such as octreotide. Octreotide treatment is associated with good clinical response in the majority of treated infants, and the medication is safe, when close clinical observation about the side effects is ensured. There are slight differences in opinions about the maximal intravenous dose of octreotide (10 or 12 μg/kg/h), but they are not clinically significant. Surgical treatment and chemical pleurodesis should be reserved for more resistant cases and should be performed in experienced pediatric surgical departments.

Author details

Ralitza Gueorguieva
Neonatal Intensive Care Unit, University Pediatric Hospital, Sofia, Bulgaria

*Address all correspondence to: raligeorgi@yahoo.com

References

[1] Rocha G. Pleural effusion in the neonate. Current Opinion in Pulmonary Medicine. 2007;**13**:305-311

[2] Long WA, Lawson EE, Harned JRHS, Kraybill EN. Pleural effusions in the first day of live: A prospective study. American Journal of Perinatology. 1984;**1**:190-194

[3] Rocha G, Fernandes P, Rocha P. Pleural effusions in the neonate. Acta Paediatrica. 2006;**95**:791

[4] Shih YT, Hua SP, Jia-Yuh C, et al. Common etiologies of neonatal pleural effusion in one third of the cases. Pediatrics and Neonatology. 2011;**52**:251-255

[5] Church JT, Antunez AG, Dean A, et al. Evidence-based management of chylothorax in infants. Journal of Pediatric Surgery. 2017;**52**:907

[6] Hansen TN, Corbet A, Ballard RA. Disorders of the chest wall, pleural cavity and diaphragm. In: Taeusch HW, Ballard AR, Gleason CA, editors. Avery s Disease of the Newborn. 8th ed. Philadelphia: Elsevier Saunders; 2005. pp. 759-778

[7] Bellini C, Odaka A, Honda N, Baba K, et al. Pulmonary sequestraktion. Journal of Pediatric Surgery. 2006;**41**:2096

[8] Thiebault DW, Zalles C, Wickstrom E. Familial pulmonary lymphatic hypoplasia associated with fetal pleural effusions. The Journal of Pediatrics. 1995;**127**:979

[9] Beigelman A, Marks KA, Landau D. Congenital isolated pleural effusion associated with obstructive uropathy. The Israel Medical Association Journal. 2005;7:271

[10] Lee C, Fang CC, Chou HC, Tsau YK. Urinothorax associated with VURD syndrome. Pediatric Nephrology. 2005;**20**:543

[11] Reitter A, Peters J, Wittelkindt B, et al. Prenatal management of fetal rhabdomyosarcoma presenting with fetal hydrops. Ultrasound in Obstetrics & Gynecology. 2012;**40**:235

[12] Odaka A, Takahashi S, Tanimizu T, et al. Chest wall mesenchymal hamartoma associated with massive fetal pleural effusion: A case report. Journal of Pediatric Surgery. 2005;**40**:e5

[13] Ozkan H, Gulen H, Demir N, et al. Nonimmune hydrops fetalis and bilateral pulmonary hypoplasia in a newborn infant with nuchal vascular hamartoma. The Turkish Journal of Pediatrics. 1997;**39**:557

[14] Gobbi D, Rubino M, Chiandetti L, et al. Neonatal intrapericardial teratoma: A challenge for the pediatric surgeon. Journal of Pediatric Surgery. 2007;**42**:E3

[15] Longaker MT, Laberge JM, Dauserean J, Langer JC, Crombleholme TM, Callen PW, et al. Primary fetal hydrothorax: Natural history and management. Journal of Pediatric Surgery. 1989;**24**:573-576

[16] Geeta G, Singh J, Rattan KN, Bhala K. Nonchylous idiopathic pleural effusion in the newborn. Indian Journal of Critical Care Medicine. 2011;**15**(1):46-48

[17] Chernick V, Reed MH. Pneumothorax and chylothorax in the neonatal period. The Journal of Pediatrics. 1970;**76**:624-632

[18] Loukmasari A, Trialmas J, Taquim W, Pramana C. Massive pleural effusion as rare manifestation in severe neonatal sepsis. Open Access Macedonian Journal of Medical Sciences. 2021;**9**:6

[19] Armanpoor P, Armanpoor P. Neonatal pleural effusion due to COVID-19 pneumonia. Pediatrics and Neonatology. 2022;**63**(3):322-323

[20] Gupta R, Faridi MM, Gupta P. Neonatal empyema thoracis. Indian Journal of Pediatrics. 1996;**63**:704-706

[21] Proesmans M, Boeck KD. Clinical practice: Treatment of childhood empyema. European Journal of Pediatrics. 2009;**168**:639-645

[22] Mery CM, Moffett BS, Khan MS, et al. Incidence and treatment of chylothorax after cardiac surgery in children: Analysis of a large multi-institution data base. The Journal of Thoracic and Cardiovascular Surgery. 2014;**147**:678

[23] Buttiker V, Fanconi S, Burger R. Chylothorax in children: Guidelines for diagnosis and management. Chest. 1999;**116**:682-687

[24] Tutor JD, Dublin PJ, King IN, Gallagher PG. Congenital chylothorax. Current Opinion in Pediatrics. 2000;**12**:505-509

[25] Beghetti M, La Scala G, Belli D, Bugmann P, Kalangos A, Le Coultre C. Etiology and management of pediatric chylothorax. The Journal of Pediatrics. 2000;**136**(5):653-658

[26] Chan SY, Lau W, Wong WH, Cheng LC, Chau AK, Cheung YF. Chylothorax in children after congenital heart surgery. The Annals of Thoracic Surgery. 2006;**82**(5):1650-1656

[27] Pinto E, Dori Y, Smith C, et al. Neonatal lymphatic flow disorders: Impact of lymphatic imaging and interventions on outcome. Journal of Perinatology. 2021;**41**:494

[28] Costa KM, Saxena AK. Surgical chylothorax in neonates: Management and outcomes. World Journal of Pediatrics. 2018;**14**:110

[29] Ohki Y, Yoshizawa Y, Watanabe M, Kuvashima N, Morikawa A. Complications of percutaneously inserted central venous catheters in Japanese neonates. Pediatrics International. 2008;**50**:636

[30] Rejjal AR, Galal MO, Nazer HM, Karim AA, Osba YA. Complications of parenteral nutrition via an umbilical vein catheter. European Journal of Pediatrics. 1993;**152**:624

[31] Been JV, Degraenwe PLY. Pleural effusion due to intraabdominal extravasation of parenteral nutrition. Pediatric Pulmonology. 2008;**43**:1033-1035

[32] Keeney SE, Richardson CJ. Extravascular extravasation of fluid as a complication of central venous lines in the neonate. Journal of Perinatology. 1995;**15**:284-288

[33] Madhavi P, Jameson R, Robinson MJ. Unilateral pleural effusion complicating central venous catheterization. Archives of Disease in Childhood. Fetal and Neonatal Edition. 2000;**82**:F248-F249

[34] Wolthuis A, Landewe RB, ThennissenPH,WesterhuisLW.Chylothorax or leakage of total parenteral nutrition. The European Respiratory Journal. 1998;**12**:1233-1235

[35] Thakur A, Fursule A. Lung ultrasound in neonates – An underused

tool. Journal of Medical Imaging and Radiation Oncology. 2023;**67**:54

[36] McGrath EE, Blades Z, Anderson PB. Chylothorax: Etiology, diagnosis and therapeutic options. Respiratory Medicine. 2010;**104**:1-81

[37] Tutor JD. Chylothorax in infants and children. Pediatrics. 2014;**133**(4):722-733

[38] Senarathne U, Rodrigo R, Dayanath BKTP. Milky pleural effusion in a neonate and approach to investigating chylothorax. BML Case Reports. 2021;**14**:e245576. DOI: 10.1136/bcr-2021-245576

[39] Bialkowski A, Poets CF, Franz AR, et al. Congenital chylothorax: A prospective nationwide epidemiological study in Germany. Archives of Disease in Childhood. Fetal and Neonatal Ed. 2015;**100**:F169-F172

[40] Downie L, Sasi A, Malkotra A. Congenital chylothorax associations and neonatal outcomes. Journal of Paediatrics and Child Health. 2014;**50**:234-238

[41] Size SWP, Ng PC, Lam HS. Life threatening hemolytic anemia after intrapleural instillation of OK-432 for treatment of comgenital chylothorax. Neonatology. 2016;**110**:33-686

[42] White MK, Bhat R. Greenough a neonatal chylothoraces: 10 year experience in a tertiary neonatal referral centre. Case Reports in Pediatrics. 2019;**2019**:1-4

[43] Van Straaten HL, Gerards LJ, Krediet TG. Chylothorax in the neonatal period. European Journal of Pediatrics. 1993;**152**:2-5

[44] Stewart C, Linner H. Chylothorax in the newborn infant: A report of a case. American Journal of Diseases of Children. 1926;**31**:654-656

[45] Defoort P, Thiery M. Antenatal diagnosis of congenital chylothorax by gray scale sonography. Journal of Clinical Ultrasound. 1928;**6**:47-48

[46] Caserio S, Gallego C, Martin P, et al. Congenital chylothorax from fetal life to adolescence. Acta Paediatrica. 2010;**99**:1571

[47] Caserio KC, Kraver RD. Neonatal pleural effusion. Spontaneous chylothorax in a newborn with trisomy 21. Archives of Pathology & Laboratory Medicine. 2006;**130**:e22

[48] Schluter G, Steckel M, Schiffmankln H, et al. Prenatal DNA diagnosis of Noonan syndrome in a fetus with massive hygroma colli, pleural effusion and ascites. Prenatal Diagnosis. 2005;**25**:574

[49] Agrawal V, Sahin SA. Lipid pleural effusions. The American Journal of the Medical Sciences. 2008;**335**:16-20

[50] Prasad R, Singh K, Singh R. Bilateral congenital chylothorax with Noonan syndrome. Indian Pediatrics. 2002;**39**:975

[51] Bialkowski G-AJK, Zimmermann SL, Hinton RB, et al. Tetrasomy 15q25.2-qter identified with SNP microarray in a patient with multiple anomalies including complex cardiovascular malformation. American Journal of Medical Genetics. Part A. 2012;**158A**:1971

[52] Smets K. X-linked myotubular myopathy and chylothorax. Neuromuscular Disorders. 2008;**18**:183-184

[53] Lo IF, Brewer C, Shannon N, et al. Severe neonatal manifestations of

Costello syndrome. Journal of Medical Genetics. 2008;**45**:167

[54] Matsumoto N, Gondo K, Kukita J, et al. A case of galactosialidosis with a homozygous Q49R point mutation. Brain Development. 2008;**30**:595

[55] Resch B, Yildiz GS, Reiterer F. Congenital chylothorax of the newborn: Systematic analysis of published cases between 1990 and 2018. Respiration. 2022;**101**(1):84-96

[56] Krishnamorthy B, Malhotra A. Congenital chylothorax: Current perspectives and trends. Research and Reports in Neonatology. 2017;**7**:53-63

[57] Brodszki N, Lansberg JK, Dictor M, et al. A novel treatment approach for paediatric Gorham-stout syndrome with chylothorax. Acta Paediatrica. 2011;**100**(11):1448-1453

[58] Huang XZ, Wu JF. Fernando R et al fatal bilateral hydrothorax in mice lacking the integrin alpha9beta1. Molecular and Cellular Biology. 2000;**20**(14):5208-5215

[59] Ma GC, Liu CS, Chang SP, et al. A recurrent ITGA9 missence mutation in human fetuses with severe chylothorax: Possible correlation with poor response to fetal therapy. Prenatal Diagnosis. 2008;**28**(11):1058-1063

[60] Bellini C, Boccardo F, Campisi C, Bonioli E. Congenital pulmonary lymhangiectasia. Orphanet Journal of Rare Diseases. 2006;**1**:43

[61] Dutheil P, Lerailler J,Guillemette J, Wallach D. Generalized lymphangiomatosis with chylothorax and skin lymphangiomas in a neonate. Pediatric Dermatology. 1998;**15**:296

[62] Stevenson DA, Pysher TJ, Ward RM, Carey JC. Familial congenital non-immune hydrops, chylothorax and pulmonary lymphangiectasia. American Journal of Medical Genetics. 2006;**140**:368

[63] Soto Martinez M, Massie J. Chylothorax: Diagnosis and management in children. Paediatric Respiratory Reviews. 2009;**10**(4):199-207

[64] Teba L, Dedhia HV, Bowen R, Alexander JC. Chylothorax review. Critical Care Medicine. 1985;**13**(1):49-52

[65] Hillerdal G. Chylothorax and pseudochylothorax. European Respiratory Journal. 1997;**10**:1157-1162

[66] Ferguson M, Shahinian H, Michelassi F. Lymphatic smooth muscle responses to leucotriens, histamine and platelet activating factor. The Journal of Surgical Research. 1988;**44**(2):172-177

[67] Mohan H, Paes ML, Haynes S. Use of intravenous immunoglobulins as an adjunct in the conservative management of chylothorax. Paediatric Anaesthesia. 1999;**9**:89

[68] Orange JS, Geha RS, Bonilla FA. Acute chylothorax in children& selective retention of memory T-cells and natural killer cells. The Journal of Pediatrics. 2003;**143**:243

[69] Hoscote AU, Ramaiah RN, Cale CM, et al. Role of immunoglobulin supplement for secondary immunodeficiency, associated with chylothorax after pediatric cardiothoracic surgery. Pediatric Critical Care Medicine. 2012;**13**:535

[70] Al Tawil K, Ahmed G, Al-Hathal M, Al-Jarallah Y, Campbell N. Congenital chylothorax. American Journal of Perinatology. 2000;**17**(3):121-126

[71] De Beer HG, Van Straaten HL, Gerards LJ, Krediet TG. Chylothorax in

the neonatal period. European Journal of Pediatrics. 1993;**152**(1):2-5

[72] Abrams ME, Meredith KS, Kinnard P, Clark RH. Hydrops foetalis: A retrospective review of cases reported to a large national database and identification of risk factors associated with death. Pediatrics. 2007;**120**:84-89

[73] Ayida GA, Soothil PW, Rodeck CH. Survival in non-immune hydrops foetalis without malformations or chromosomal abnormalities after invasive treatment. Fetal Diagnosis and Therapy. 1995;**10**:101-105

[74] De Hann TR, Oepkes D, Beersma MF, et al. Aetiology, diagnosis and treatment of hydrops foetalis. Current Pediatric Reviews. 2005;**1**:63-72

[75] Fahnenstich H, Schmid G, Havercamp F, et al. Non-immune hydrops foetalis – An analysis of liveborn cases. Pediatric Reviews and Communications. 1992;**6**:231-224

[76] Greenough A, Roberton NR. Acute respiratory distress in the newborn. In: Rennie JM, Roberton NR, editors. Textbook of Neonatology. 3rd ed. London: Churchill Livingston; 1999. pp. 481-607

[77] Wadhwa S, Verma M, Kaur J. Pleural effusion in neonatal period. A case report. Indian Pediatrics. 1976;**13**:729-731

[78] BA MGS, Ellefson RD, Budahn LL, et al. The lipoprotein profile of chylous and non chylous pleural effusions. Mayo Clinic Proceedings. 1980;**55**:700-704

[79] Hooper C, Lee YCG, Maskell N, et al. Investigation of unilateral pleural effusion in adults: British Thoracic Society pleural disease guideline 2010. Thorax. 2010;**65**(Suppl. 2):ii 4-ii17

[80] Maldonado F, Hawkins FJ, Daniels CE, et al. Pleural fluid characteristics of chylothorax. Mayo Clinic Proceedings. 2009;**84**:129-133

[81] Ahmed AAH, Yacoub TE. Empyema thoracis. Clinical Medicine Insights. Circulatory, Respiratory and Pulmonary Medicine. 2010;**4**:1-8

[82] Lee CJ, Tsao PN, Chen CY, Hsieh WS, Liou JY, Chou HC. Prenatal therapy improves the survival of premature infants with congenital chylothorax. Pediatrics and Neonatology. 2016;**57**(2):127-132

[83] Bartha JL, Comino-Delgado R. Fetal chylothorax response to maternal dietary treatment. Obstetrics and gynaecology. 2001;**97**(5 pt 2):820-823

[84] Chen C, Chang T, Wang W. Resolution of bilateral fetal chylothorax and ascites afterafter two unilateral thoracocentesis. Ultrasound in Obstetrics & Gynecology. 2001;**18**:401-406

[85] Dendale G, Comet P, Amram D, et al. Le chylothorax de decouverte antenatale. Archives de Pédiatrie. 1999;**6**(8):867-871

[86] Picone O, Benachi A, Mandelbrot L, Ruano R, Dumez Y, Dommergues M. Thoracoamniotic shunting for fetal pleural effusions with hydrops. American Journal of Obstetrics and Gynecology. 2004;**191**(6):2047-2050

[87] Okawa T, Takano Y, Fujimori K, Yanagida K, Sato A. A new fetal therapy for chylothorax: Pleurodesis with OK-432. Ultrasound in Obstetrics & Gynecology. 2001;**18**(4):376-377

[88] Tanemura M, Nishikawa N, Kojima K, Suzuki Y, Suzumori K. A case of successful fetal therapy for congenital chylothorax by intrapleural injection of OK-432. Ultrasound in Obstetrics & Gynecology. 2001;**18**(4):371-375

[89] Jorgensen C, Brocks V, Bang J, Jorgensen FS, Ronsbro L. Treatment of severe fetal chylothorax associated with pronounced hydrops with intrapleural injection of OK-432. Ultrasound in Obstetrics & Gynecology. 2003;**21**(1):66

[90] Tsukihara A, Tanemura M, Suzuki Y, Sato T, Tanaka T, Suzumori K. Reduction of pleural effusion by OK-432 in a fetus complicated with congenital hydrothorax. Fetal Diagnosis and Therapy. 2004;**19**(4):327-331

[91] Rodeck CH, Fisk NM, Fraser DI, et al. Long term in utero drainage of fetal hydrothorax. The New England Journal of Medicine. 1988;**319**(17):1135-1138

[92] Mallmann M, Graham V, Rosing B, et al. Thoracoamniotic shunting for fetal hydrothorax: Predictors of intrauterine course and postnatal outcome. Fetal Diagnosis and Therapy. 2017;**41**:58-65

[93] Mussat P, Dommergues M, Parat S, et al. Congenital chylothorax with hydrops: Postnatal care and outcome following antenatal diagnosis. Acta Paediatrica. 1995;**84**(7):749-755

[94] Nicolaides KH, Azar GB. Thoraco-amniotic shunting. Fetal Diagnosis and Therapy. 1990;**5**(3-4):153-164

[95] Smith RP, Illanes P, Denbow ML, et al. Outcome of fetal pleural effusions treated by thoracoamniotic shunting. Ultrasound in Obstetrics & Gynecology. 2005;**26**(1):63-66

[96] Thompson PJ, Greenough A, Nicolaides KH. Respiratory function in infancy following pleuro-amniotic shunting. Fetal Diagnosis and Therapy. 1993;**8**(2):79-83

[97] Williams KR, Burford TH. The management of chylothorax. Annals of Surgery. 1964;**160**:131-140

[98] Sepulveda W, Galindo A, Sosa A, Diaz L, Flores X, de la Fuente P. Intrathoracic dislodgement of pleuro-amniotic shunt. Three case reports with long term follow-up. Fetal Diagnosis and Therapy. 2005;**20**(2):102-105

[99] Chen M, Hsiey C, Shih JC, et al. Proinflammatory migratory inhibition factor and interleukin –6 are concentrated in pleural effusion of human fetuses with prenatal chylothorax. Prenatal Diagnosis. 2007;**27**:435-441

[100] Chen M, Chen CP, Shih JC, et al. Antenatal treatment of chylothorax and cystic hygroma with OK-432 in non-immune hydrops foetalis. Fetal Diagnosis and Therapy. 2005;**20**(4):309-315

[101] Yang YS, MaGC SJC, et al. Experimental treatment of bilateral fetal chylothorax using in utero pleurodesis. Ultrasound in Obstetrics & Gynecology. 2012;**39**:56-62

[102] Parra J, Amenedo M, Muniz-Diaz E, Ormo F, Simo M, Vega C. A new successful therapy for fetal chylothorax by intrapleural injection of maternal blood. Ultrasound in Obstetrics & Gynecology. 2003;**22**:290-293

[103] Philips JB, Atkinson TP. Management of chronic pleural effusions in the neonate. In: Martin R, section editor. Up to Date. 12 May 2023

[104] Biewer ES, Zurn C, Arnold R, et al. Chylotjorax after surgery on congenital heart disease in newborn and infants – risk factors and efficacy of MCT – diet. Journal of Cardiothoracic Surgery. 2010;**5**:127

[105] Shih YT, Su PH, Chen JY, et al. Common etiologies of neonatal pleural effusions. Pediatrics and Neonatology. 2011;**52**:251

[106] Chan GM, Lichtenberg E. The use of fat free human milk in infants with chylous pleural effusion. Journal of Perinatology. 2007;**27**:434

[107] Young S, Dalgleish S, Eccleston A, Akierman A, McMillan D. Severe congenital chylothorax treated with octreotide. Journal of Perinatology. 2004;**24**(3):200-202

[108] Glaser B, Hirsch HJ, Landau H. Persistent hyperinsulinemic hypoglycemia of infancy: Long-term octreotide treatment without pancreatectomy. The Journal of Pediatrics. 1993;**123**(4):644-650

[109] Rasiah SV, Oei J, Lui K. Octreotide in the treatment of congenital chylothorax. Journal of Paediatrics and Child Health. 2004;**40**(9-10):585-588

[110] Das A, Shah P. Octreotide for the treatment of chylothorax in neonates. Cochrane Data Base Systemic Review. 2010;**9**:CD006388

[111] Reck-Burneo CA, Parekh A, Velcek FT. Is octreotide a risk factor for necrotizing enterocolitis? Journal of Pediatric Surgery. 2008;**43**(6):1209-1210

[112] Averalo RP, Bullabh P, Krauss AN, et al. Octreotide induced hypoxemia and pulmonary hypertension in premature neonates. Journal of Pediatric Surgery. 2005;**38**(2):251-253

[113] Goto M, Kawamata K, Kitano M, Watanabe K, Chiba J. Treatment of chylothorax in a premature infant using somatostatin. Journal of Perinatology. 2003;**23**:563-564

[114] Cleveland K, Zook D, Harvey K, Woods RK. Massive chylothorax in small babies. Journal of Pediatric Surgery. 2009;**44**:546-550

[115] Cannizzaro V, Frey B, Bernet–Buettiker V, The role of somatostatin in the treatment of persistent chylothorax in children, European Journal of Cardio-Thoracic Surgery, 2006; 30; 49-53

[116] Horvers M, Mooij CF, Antonius TA. Is octreotide treatment useful in patients with congenital chylothorax in newborns. Neonatology. 2012;**101**:225

[117] Bellini C, Cabano R, De Angelis LC, et al. Octreotide for congenital and acquired chylothorax in newborns: A systematic review. Journal of Paediatrics and Child Health. 2018;**58**:840

[118] Mizuno T, Fukuda T, Emoto C, et al. Developmental pharmacokinetics of sirolimus: Implications for precision dosing in neonates and infants with complicated vascular anomalies. Pediatric Blood & Cancer. 2017;**64**(8):e26470

[119] Liviskie CJ, Brennan CC, McPherson CC, Vesoulis ZA. Propranolol for the treatment of lymphatic malformations in the neonate – A case report and review of literature. Journal of Pediatric Pharmacology and Therapeutics. 2020;**25**:155

[120] Mitchell K, Weiner A, Ramsay P, Sahni M. Use of propranolol in the treatment of chylous effusions in infants. Pediatrics. 2021;**148**(1):e2020049699

[121] Handal-Orefice R, Midura D, Wu JK, et al. Propranolol therapy for congenital chylothorax. Pediatrics. 2023;**151**(2):e2022058555

[122] Matsukuma E, Aoki Y, Sakai M, et al. Treatment with OK-432 for persistent congenital chylothorax in newborn infants resistant to octreotide. Journal of Pediatric Surgery. 2009;**44**:e37

[123] Kamiyama M, Usui N, Tani G, et al. Postoperative chylothorax in congenital diaphragmatic hernia. European Journal of Pediatric Surgery. 2010;**20**:391

[124] Scottoni F, Fusaro F, Conforti A, et al. Pleurodesis with povidone-jodine for refractory chylothorax in newborns: Personal experience and literature review. Journal of Pediatric Surgery. 2015;**50**:1722

[125] Mitanchez D, Walter-Nicolet E, Salomon R, et al. Congenital chylothorax: What is the best strategy. Archives of Disease in Childhood. Fetal and Neonatal Edition. 2006;**91**:F53

[126] Hoff DS, Gremmels DB, Hall KM, et al. Dosage and effectiveness of intrapleural doxycycline for pediatric postcardiotomy pleural effusions. Pharmacotherapy. 2007;**27**:995

[127] Antony VB, Rorhfuss KJ, Godbey SW, Sparks JA, Hott JW. Mechanism of tetracycline-hydrochloride induced pleurodesis. Tetracycline – Hydrochloride stimulated mesothelial cells growth factor-like activity for fibroblasts. American Review of Respiratory Disease. 1992;**146**(4):1009-1013

[128] Utture A, Kodur V, Mondkar J. Chemical pleurodesis with oxytetracycline in congenital chylothorax. Indian Pediatrics. 2016;**53**(12):1105-1106

[129] Hodges MM, Crombleholme TM, Meyers M, et al. Massive fetal chylothorax successfully treated with postnatal talc pleurodesis: A case report and review of the literature. Journal of Pediatric Surgery Case Reports. 2016;**9**(Suppl. C):1-4

[130] Faul JL, Berry GJ, Colby TV, Ruoss SJ, Walter MB, Rosen GD. Thoracic lymphangiomas, lymphangiectasis, lymphangiomatosis and lymphatic dysplasia syndroms. American Journal of Respiratory and Critical Care Medicine. 2000;**161**:1037-1046

[131] Resch B, Halmer M, Muller WD, Eber E. Long term follow-up of children with congenital chylothorax. The European Respiratory Journal. 2012;**40**:1060-1062

Chapter 2

Surgical Treatment of Pleural Empyema in Children

Iván Alcoholado Boye

Abstract

Pleural empyema is a common infectious pathology in pediatrics that requires timely treatment to achieve ad integrum recovery. The clinical understanding of the pathophysiological evolution of the disease and the knowledge of the methods of its imaging study allow the treating physician to add to the antibiotic treatment, such as drainage of the pleural space and/or thoracoscopy that has historically been performed. In recent years, many centers have replaced it with intrapleural injection of fibrinolytics with good results. Drainage and minimally invasive surgery procedures are detailed. The aim of the chapter is that the student has a comprehensive knowledge of the treatment and to keep in mind that both early diagnosis and timely treatment prevent the progressing of the disease and its possible complications.

Keywords: parapneumonic effusion, loculated parapneumonic effusion, pleural empyema, surgical treatment, fibrinolytics

1. Introduction

The visceral pleura covers the lung and the parietal pleura covers the inner wall of the hemithorax, leaving a virtual space between both, which in normal conditions houses between 0.1 and 0.2 ml/kg of pleural fluid with physical-chemical characteristics that serves as a lubricant for the pleural surfaces moving. The blood supply to the parietal pleura is from the arteries' superior intercostals and phrenics and that of the visceral does of the pulmonary and pericardiophrenic arteries; some areas may be supplied by bronchial arteries. Venous drainage from the visceral pleura goes to the pulmonary veins and that of the parietal to the intercostal veins. The pleural lymphatics drain to supra and infradiaphragmatic networks. The flow of pleural fluid is regulated by Starling's law which influences the hydrostatic and osmotic pressure of the pleural liquid. Under normal conditions, it can be renewed up to 500 ml of pleural fluid per day in a permanent active balance of transport and purification, in adults. In children, a production of 2 ml/hour in each hemithorax, has been noted. Pleural fluid accumulates when a disturbance occurs on the gradient between hydrostatic and oncotic pressure [1, 2].

The parapneumonic effusions are the result of the spread of inflammation to the pleura with the consequent accumulation of proteins, fluids and leukocytes in the pleural space forming the spill. Small amounts of protein are removed easily by the lymphatic system but when they increase as occurs in pneumonia due to increased capillary permeability, the lymphatic system is insufficient, producing the spill pleural. Initially, the pleural effusion is sterile with a low count of leukocytes. Over the hours or days, the bacteria invade the fluid, and the effusion can become thick and fibrotic resulting in empyema, which is defined as the presence of purulent fluid in the pleural cavity. The risk of developing a true pleural empyema is determined by a balance between the host resistance, bacterial virulence and timing presentation for medical treatment [1, 2].

The aim of the chapter is to analyze a common infectious pathology in pediatrics that may require various medical-surgical treatments. To achieve a good understanding of the topic, the definitions will be indicated according to the pathophysiological evolution of the disease and the study methods that will allow deciding the best complementary therapeutic alternative to antibiotics, from pleurodesis, drainage of the pleural space to minimally minimal surgery invasive that will be detailed, so that you can be put into practice. The non-thoracoscopic alternative of treatment with fibrinolytics that is used in many centers will also be taught and finally, the possible complications that, unfortunately, are not exempt from the treatment of pleural empyema will be indicated.

2. Definition

Pleural empyema is defined as the accumulation of fluid infected in the pleural space. Empyema derived from the Greek word empyein which means to "put pus in." The most common infectious agents are bacteria, but they also may be caused by viral, fungal and *Mycoplasma pneumoniae*. Much less commonly can also result from chest trauma, post thoracic surgery, esophageal perforation or extension of an infection retropharyngeal, mediastinal, paravertebral, abdominal and retroperitoneal spaces, especially in immunocompromised children [1, 2].

An inflammation or an infection within or adjacent to the pleural space, rarely resolves spontaneously because host defenses are limited by the anatomy and physiology of the pleural space [3–5].

2.1 Definitions relation to pleural effusions/empyema

- Pleural effusions in general can be of two types depending on the underlying pathology: transudative effusion that is produced by an imbalance between hydrostatic and oncotic pressure in different pathologies, unlike parapneumonic effusion, which is an exudative effusion. Represents an alteration of factors localities that lead to an accumulation of pleural fluid. Initially, this pleural effusion is free-flowing and sterile.

- Pleural empyema is defined macroscopically by the presence of cloudy purulent fluid, frank pus or fibrinopus in the pleural cavity. Microscopically, when the study of the pleural fluid that is carried out immediately in the microbiology laboratory shows bacteria in the Gram stain and when the seeding of the fluid by the laboratory shows germs in the culture, the result of which takes hours or days depending on the different techniques used and type of germ.

- Complicated parapneumonic effusion corresponds when the initial exudate changes due to the invasion of germs in the pleural space or when the proteins increase and coagulate forming septa that loculate said space, causing greater accumulation of fluid. As the child has usually been treated with antibiotics to treat pneumonia and the defensive mechanisms eliminate the bacteria or pass them into the lymphatic circulation network, cultures of the fluid are usually negative.

- Loculated parapneumonic effusion refers to the presence of septations within the effusion, which interfere with the free flow of fluid. Loculations are caused by the accumulation of proteinaceous debris in the fluid as the disease progresses and can be detected by imaging ultrasonography.

- Complicated pneumonia refers to pneumonia with any complication, including in different percentages loculated parapneumonic effusion, empyema, necrotizing pneumonia, parenchymal cavitations, bronchiopleura fistula, pneumothorax or lung abscess.

3. History

After the Second World War, a commission was formed to study the cause of the high mortality from cadres' respiratory problems among soldiers and how to avoid it. The call Graham Commission, in 1918, concluded that: "the infected liquid in the pleural space must be completely drained: early with closed methods and late, surgical drainage is more effective" and that "chronic empyema is avoided by early treatment of the infected pleural space" [2], what is valid to date.

4. Epidemiology

Parapneumonic effusion/empyema develops in 2–12%of children with pneumonia and in up to 28%of children requiring hospitalization [6, 7] and on the other hand, between 75 and 95% of cases of empyema are the result of pneumonia complicated by infected. It is most common among young children; rates are 3.7, 3.9 and 1.3 cases per 100,000 population among children under 2 years, 2 to 4 years and 5 to 17 years, respectively. Males and females are equally affected [6]. The mortality rate is low but may be higher in infants [6, 7]. Most deaths are due to the acute pneumonia or sepsis rather than the pleural disease.

Certain underlying diseases may increase the risk of parapneumonic effusion/empyema in children. In one review of 61 children with parapneumonic effusion/empyema, 11%had an underlying illness or condition [8]. Predisposing problems include immunodeficiencies [7–10], influenza [11], malignancy [8], Down syndrome [7, 9], congenital thrombocytopenia [8], cerebral palsy [7–9], prior surgery [8, 12, 13] tuberculosis [10], congenital heart disease [7], prematurity [7], history of esophageal stricture [7, 8] and cystic fibrosis [7].

The bacteriology of infected pleural fluid has varied with the introduction of antibiotics, the development of resistance to them and the widespread use of vaccines for *Haemophilus influenzae* type B and *Streptococcus pneumoniae* [14]. Unfortunately, 35–46% of children do not achieve to identify etiological agents in the culture. In a review by Strong Memorial Hospital - University of Rochester, New York between 1962 and 1980, empyema was reported in approximately 0.6% of children with bacterial pneumonia, despite diagnosis and treatment [15]. However, the number of children with parapneumonic is increasing as demonstrated prospective studies of pneumonia acquired in the community [7]. Some other less common bacteria are being identified as a cause of empyema, such as Streptococcus viridans [16], Streptococcus group A and Actinomyces sp. [17]. The beta-hemolytic Streptococcus A infection associated with empyema and septic shock syndrome has been reported as a complication of chickenpox, immunodeficiency and rarely in healthy children [18]. In Chile, in the Pediatric Service of the Clinical Hospital of the Pontifical Catholic University of Chile, cultures were made in 24 children with pleural empyema, achieving a bacteriological yield in 15 (63%) and of these the *Streptococcus pneumoniae* was the most frequent with 60% of cases [19]. Empyema occurs twice as frequently in winter/spring than in summer/autumn and the mortality rate is higher in the children under 2 years [6].

In relation to pleural empyema during the recent Covid-19 pandemic there are already several interesting reports in world literature. In Hong Kong, in the post-COVID-19 period, a marked decrease in the incidence of pleural empyema in children was observed, while the incidence in adults remained similar. Polymicrobial etiology increased while *Streptococcus pneumoniae* etiology decreased. The authors postulate that this is related to the delay of children with pneumonia in going to the hospital [20]. In Australia, social distancing measures instituted due to #SARSCoV2 dramatically reduced cases of pleural empyema in children, according to the authors [21]. In the Netherlands, the increase in notifiable invasive group A streptococcal (iGAS) infections doubled between July 2021 and June 2022 compared to before COVID-19. There was a strong increase, more pronounced in children under 5 years of age and for the diagnoses of pleural empyema and necrotizing fasciitis. As the authors note, this increase in pediatric iGAS warrants investigation and surveillance [22].

Despite pediatric pleural empyema being included in the International Classification of Diseases, 10th Revision, Clinical Modification or Procedure Coding System (ICD-10-CM/PCS), there is no comparative literature on smoking, obese or diabetic children with pleural empyema compared to previously healthy children who develop pleural empyema [23].

Studies in adults show that in patients with empyema, the rate of smokers and diabetics exceeded the average rate of the general population of smokers and diabetic patients [24].

Studies in adult diabetics with pleural empyema indicate that the time to lung expansion after operation was longer. Stricter pre- and post-operative control of blood-sugar levels and adequate antibiotics are required to facilitate postoperative lung re-expansion. In patients with thickened pleurae, prolonged chest tube placement is unavoidable [25].

5. Etiology

Parapneumonic effusion/empyema in children occurs primarily in association with underlying bacterial pneumonia. *Streptococcus pneumoniae* (pneumococcus), community-acquired *Staphylococcus aureus* including methicillin-resistant *S. aureus* [MRSA] and group A Streptococcus are the predominant causative organisms.

Streotococcus pneumoniae (pneumococcus) has been the most common pathogen causing parapneumonic effusions and empyema, but its prevalence has decreased with the use of pneumococcal vaccines [26, 27]. The predominant causative organisms have changed over time with the advent of antibiotic therapy. The widespread use of polysaccharide and conjugate vaccines against *Haemophilus influenzae* type b2 and *Streptococcus pneumoniae* has also contributed [14].

Over a decade, in several places in the world, Methicillin-resistant *Staphylococcus aureus* has increased its frequency, and *Streptococcus pneumoniae* has invasive strain variants. Other germs such as Pseudomonas have appeared as etiological agents. It is due to the appearance of non-susceptible serotypes and multidrug-resistant phenotypes especially after the introduction of new conjugate vaccines of a broader spectrum [28–30]. To reduce resistance to antibiotics, it is necessary to strictly comply with the schemes indicated by the infectious diseases committee of each hospital, and be attentive to changes in the frequency of etiological germs and their sensitivity and the appearance of new serotypes that may be resistant.

6. Pathogeny

The pathological manifestations of the natural evolution of the pleural empyema according to the consensus of the American Thoracic Society (1962) have been divided into three phases or stages, that develop chronologically as follows:

- 1st exudative phase
- 2nd phase fibrinopurulent and
- 3rd and last phase of the process is the organization

However, prior to these states, there is always a pre-collection stage that is characterized by a localized pleuritis.

As shown in **Table 1**, the physical-chemical and bacteriological characteristics of the pleural effusion change according to the pathological phases in the natural evolution of the parapneumonic effusion that develops chronologically, if no treatment is provided.

Phase	Exudative	Fibrino purulent	Organization
Pleural fluid	Serous	Cloudy or purulent	Scant
pH	>7.3	<7.1	<7.1
Bacteria	Sterile	Present according to the use of antibiotics	Present or not according to antibiotic uses
Glycemia (mg/dl)	> 60	< 40	< 40
Units of Lactic dehydrogenase	< 500	> 1.000	> 1.000
White Blood Cells	< 1.000	> 5.000	Variable
Pleural Peel	Absent or thin elastic	Thin inelastic	Thick rigid to fibrous
Duration	24–72 hours	7–10 days	Starts in 3rd–4th week (lasts for months)

Table 1.
Physical–chemical and bacteriological characteristics of the pleural effusion according to the pathological phases in the natural evolution of the parapneumonic effusion.

6.1 Exudative phase

There is an accumulation of inflammatory fluid with characteristics of exudate, serous in appearance and generally sterile. Contains white blood cells in less than 1000 per mm3, lactic dehydrogenase with more than 500 units, the pH is greater than 7.3, glucose is between 40 and 60 mg/dl and staining of Gram no bacterial agents are found. It is a liquid easy to drain, and does not interfere with lung expansion when its volume is low. This phase can last as little as 24 to 72 hours [31].

6.2 Fibrinopurulent phase

This phase or classic empyema corresponds to a complicated parapneumonic effusion. The pleural space is infected. Fibrinogenesis occurs and fibrinolytic activity decreases. The procoagulant effect as the pH decreases, increases fibrinopus deposits on the pleurae. A matrix of septa is formed between the visceral and parietal pleura with multiple loculations. In addition, white blood cells in the pleural fluid increase.

The fluid changes characteristics of exudate to fibrinopurulent with a cloudy or purulent appearance and with the presence of germs. The physical-chemical characteristics also change: there is a greater number of white blood cells that can exceed 5.000 per mm3, lactic dehydrogenase rises above 1.000 units, the pH is more acid (which allows more coagulation of proteins), even reaching 7.1 or less and at Gram there are germs although the culture may be negative for the use of antibiotics and glucose drops to less than 40 mg/dl, for consumption as energy by bacteria. As the purulent pleural fluid becomes acidic, it thickens and septa appear that subdivide the pleural space in multiple loculations. The fibrin is deposited on the pleurae especially in decubitus areas, beginning to form a thin and inelastic fibrin peel or shell which ends up thickening and progressively restricting lung expansion, decreasing the ability to oxygen exchange in that lung, rendering it ineffective ipsilateral kinesiotherapy. Antibiotic levels are low in the pleural fluid and the physicochemical conditions make them less effective, as occurs with aminoglycosides [32, 33]. This phase can last 7 to 10 days.

6.3 Organization phase or fibrosis

If the process continues its natural course, it reaches the phase of organization or fibrosis in which the pleural fluid increasingly is less until it disappears, the leukocytes are in quantity variable, lactic dehydrogenase is also maintained at variable levels, pH remains below 7.1, glucose persists below 40 mg/dl and there may or may not be bacteria on the staining of Gram, according to the use of antibiotics.

Fibroblasts proliferate in both pleurae, producing a membrane or fibrin shell that is thicker and more rigid, known as peel. In addition, there is a large increase in newly formed capillaries between the peel or fibrous shell and the visceral pleura, between the fourth to fifth and even sixth week of initiation of the empyema. Fibrosis progressively increases until finally the lung is trapped and immobilized firmly, which prevents its normal expansion. The organizational phase or stage results in a thick cortex that can trap the lung. It is perfused but not ventilated, which manifests as chronic restrictive lung disease.

Despite being sequentially outlined, there is no certainty that each will progress to the next and on the other hand, it is important to point out that not all the pleural space is always in the same phase with the same intensity, since the dorsal decubitus and the recesses of the pleural cavity are generally areas with more compromised or advanced disease. More importantly, the stage of pleural disease may not relate to the degree of physiologic illness of a child. The severity of illness is determined by the extent of underlying parenchymal disease, the extent of intravascular inflammatory response and the extent of the impact in the pleural space of the hemithorax. Patients may be quite systemically ill early in the course of severe pneumonia but clinically later on in empyema development, which should be considered prior to intervention should always be viewed considering the layers of processes when treating empyema.

7. Clinical diagnosis

The symptoms and signs of pleural empyema are generally difficult to differentiate from those of pneumonia since it is observed fever, malaise, dyspnea, chest pain with breathing, usually productive cough and exceptionally cyanosis. Anorexia and chest pain with inspiratory stop are added that can make a difference. On physical examination the signs are also similar to those of pneumonia such as tachypnea with variable degree retraction, inspiratory stop, decrease to a greater or lesser degree of the lung murmur; in addition to crackles, tubal murmur, dullness to percussion and there may be abdominal distension from ileus which may increase respiratory distress, so it should be evaluated with a chest x-ray and abdominal x-ray if necessary [34].

Empyema should always be suspected when a child with pneumonia does not improve with antibiotic therapy, or your symptoms worsen after early signs of improvement. A significant rise in temperature, oxygen-demanding hypoxia, leukocytosis and an increase in C-reactive protein are suggestive of an infected parapneumonic pleural effusion.

8. Evaluation and study

When a child with pneumonia does not respond to antibiotic treatment within 48 hours, the possibility of a parapneumonic effusion should be considered. Since it is not always possible to determine if there is an effusion or more aggressive pneumonia during a physical examination, a chest x-ray should be used. Radiology constitutes an element of valuable help to determine the presence of occupancy of the space fluid pleural. Pleural effusions in the exudative phase or stages in children are classified as small effusion if the opacification is less than a quarter of a hemithorax, moderate if the opacification is between a quarter and a half hemithorax and large when it is more than half a hemithorax on upright radiographs [35]. Unfortunately, the standing position, which is very useful in older children, cannot be performed in small children, so we must know how to interpret the x-rays in the supine position.

As shown in **Figure 1** of an infant child in a supine position with partial opacification of the pleural space, it is not possible to determine whether the pleural effusion is septated or not. As the effusion is more than 10 millimeters thick, we complemented it with **Figure 2**, which demonstrates a liquid pleural effusion without septa, so it is free.

In chest **Figure 3** of a preschool girl in a supine position shows complete opacification of the pleural space with air bronchogram. Nor can we define whether said spill

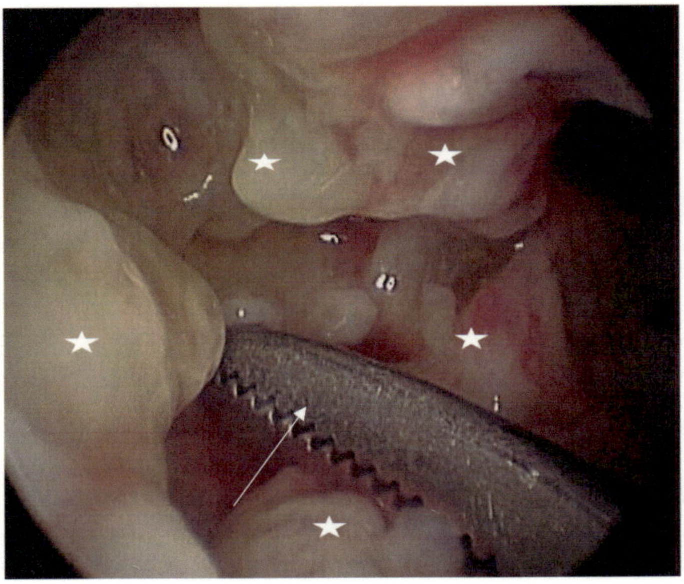

Figure 1.
Anteroposterior chest X-ray in decubitus: Moderate right pleural effusion (unfilled arrow) with intercissural effusion (single arrow).

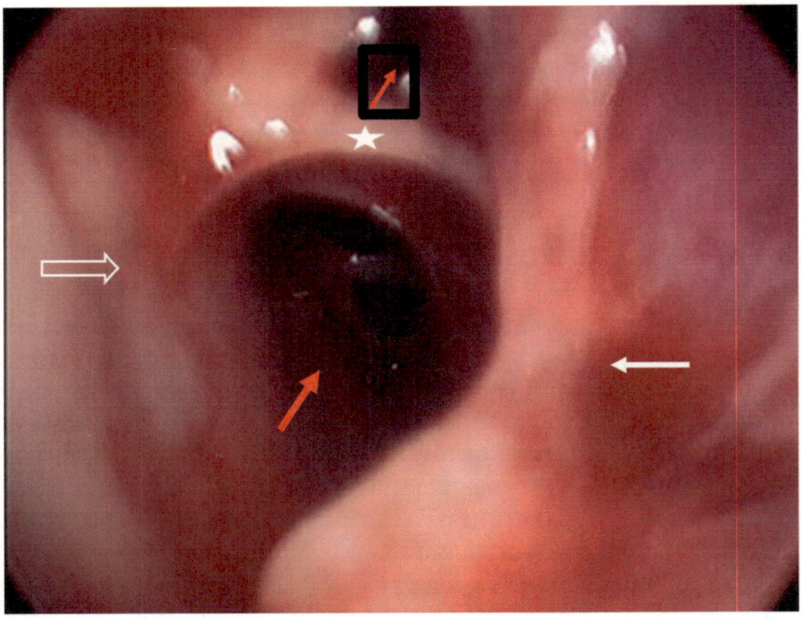

Figure 2.
*Chest ultrasound showing free pleural effusion without septations (unfilled arrow), corresponding to the patient in **Figure 1**.*

pleural is septated or not. In this scenario, it is appropriate to perform **Figure 4**, which demonstrates a pleural effusion with multiple septa with the formation of locules with heterogeneous content.

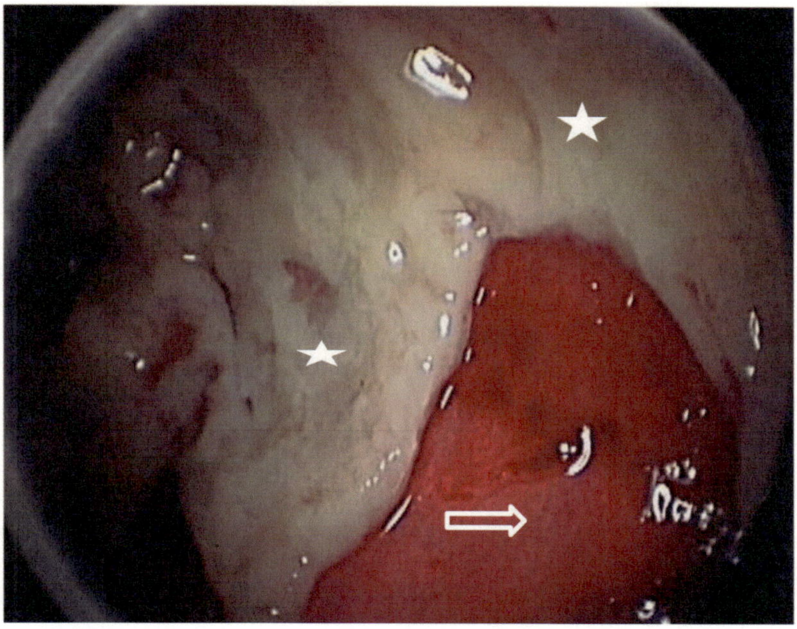

Figure 3.
Anteroposterior chest X-ray in decubitus: Complete opacification of the right hemithorax (unfilled arrow) with air bronchogram (single black arrow). Radiologically, it is not possible to clarify whether or not said pleural effusion has septations.

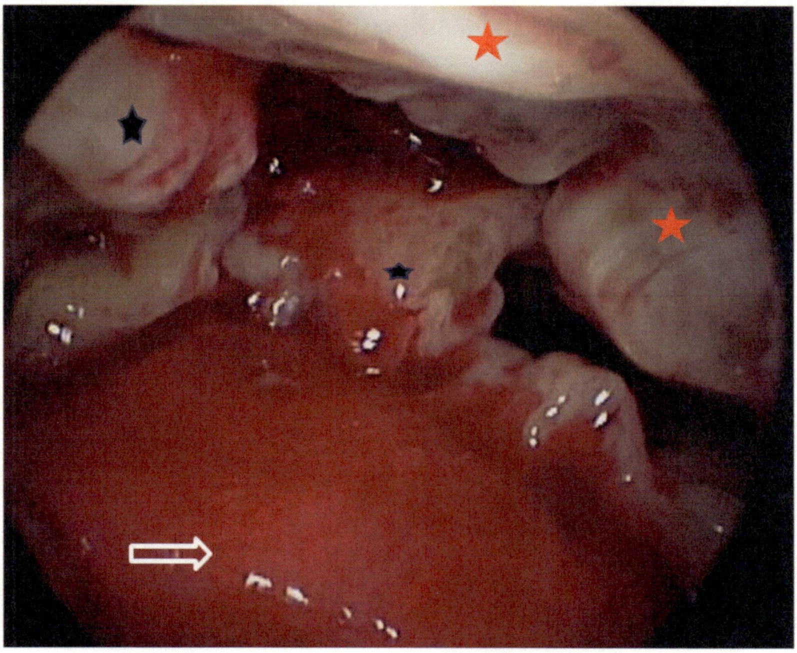

Figure 4.
*Chest ultrasound corresponding to the patient in the **Figure 3** showing pleural effusion with multiple septations (White arrow) with formation of loculations (asterisk), echoes inside (red arrow) and thickening of the visceral pleura (unfilled arrow).*

According to the distribution of the effusions in pleural space, the clinician can determine if this fluid is free or not, and thus be able to define which treatment is the most appropriate for the girl or boy which we will see in the treatment subsection.

Is it different in schoolchildren and adolescents who have had a chest x-ray taken in a standing position? If it has opacification of the pleural space with the classic Damoiseau curve we must assume that said fluid could be free in the costophrenic sinus but if the effusion does not have the typical marked curve, most likely the fluid is already septated. However, radiographs alone cannot differentiate an empyema from a parapneumonic effusion [36]. In this scenario, it is preferable to request an ultrasound of the spill, which provides excellent information. The need for chest x-rays in pleuropneumonia for diagnosis and treatment control in relation to radiation corresponds to the sum of each of them. It is not dangerous from the point of view of radiation biology unlike computed tomography [37, 38].

There is an inappropriate practice - there being the possibility of performing an ultrasound of the effusion - of performing x-rays in the lateral decubitus position with a horizontal beam to try to clarify whether the fluid is free or distributed. Unfortunately, the occupation of space pleural radiologically does not differentiate between thickening pleural, fluids and septations. If there is free liquid on the side right, for example, occupation of the space should be observed right pleural in the film in right lateral decubitus, which would have to disappear on the plate in the lateral decubitus position left. Loculated pleural effusions are usually not evident in decubitus radiographs, which can delay treatment. If on the lateral decubitus film, the radiograph shows a space occupation greater than 10 mm thick, the test of choice to continue is a chest ultrasound that allows us to see the pleural fluid, its characteristics and the presence or absence of partitions with the added advantage of being portable, relatively inexpensive and radiation-free (see **Figure 5** = Use of images for management of pleural effusion). On a stage more advanced, ultrasound allows us to see fibrin septa that form locules of variable size and content in different coagulation

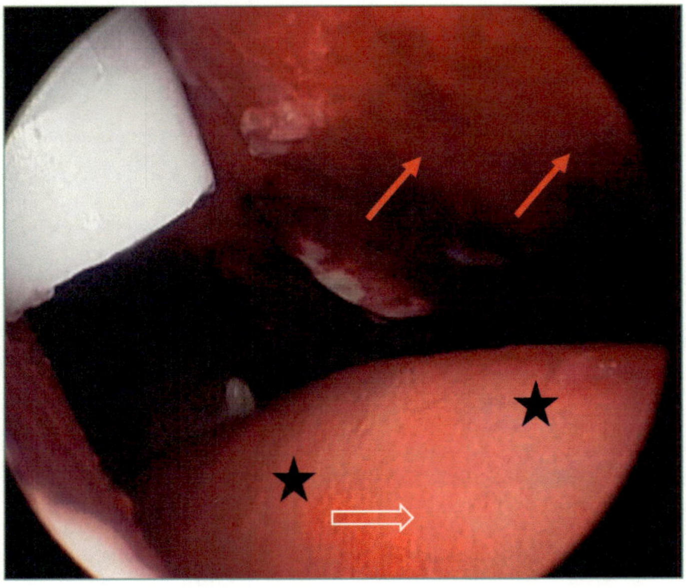

Figure 5.
Pleuropneumonia with free effusion management (low grade).

stages from semi-liquid, semi-coagulated or coagulated according to the evolution time. In addition, it allows marking the ideal puncture or drainage site and/or ultrasound guidance of the procedure to evacuate fluid and send a sample to the laboratory for study [39]. Since it has already been noted that pleural effusions are not always in the same phase throughout the pleural space, ultrasound should inspect the entire pleural space from the apex to the costophrenic and cardiophrenic sinuses.

Quite useful is the ultrasonographic classification of infectious pleural effusion, which classifies them in grades according to ultrasound characteristics of the pleural effusion. As shown in **Figure 2**, the low-grade pleural effusion is homogeneous without echoes in suspension or septa and is not associated with pleural thickening and as shown in **Figure 4**, the high-grade effusion presents echoes inside with formation of loculations and thickening of the visceral pleura [40]. This classification makes it possible to define complementary treatment behaviors to the antibiotic such as pleurocentesis, drainage or video surgery, according to the degree and volume of the effusion, as will be indicated in the subsection treatment.

Computed tomography (CT) is useful when we suspect that the condensation of the parenchyma is undergoing changes that can modify our behavior, such as necrotization late-stage pneumonia or abscess formation, but it does not allow us to specify the nature of the liquid, the presence of empyema or see the fibrin septa since these are not vascularized and therefore cannot be visualized [41]. As a result of these limitations, chest CT should not be routinely performed in the evaluation of children with parapneumonic effusions.

Blood cultures should be performed in all children with parapneumonic effusion, being positive between 10% and 22% of children with complicated effusions and are particularly useful if the culture of pleural fluid is negative [42].

Pleural fluid should be studied for analysis including Gram stain and bacterial culture; there are reports of positivity in up to 63% but most studies report culture positive in less than 25% [18].

8.1 Exudative phase

If the child has an uncomplicated parapneumonic pleural effusion (low grade) will respond to thoracentesis, sucking up liquid as much as possible (up to a maximum of 10 to 20 ml/kg) plus antibiotic [43]. If the spill cannot be adequately evacuated, if it is reproducing or if the volume of non-septate pleural fluid is greater than 1 cm on a radiograph in decubitus or the opacity is greater than a quarter of the hemithorax based on the upright film, it must be drained. This behavior will allow for improved inspiratory volume and decrease the possibility of that said effusion is septated. On the other hand, if the parapneumonic free pleural effusion is complicated from the cytochemical point of view in the sample of the pleurocentesis for presenting germs to the Gram or the pH is lower than 7.2 or glucose less than 40 mg/dl or dehydrogenase greater than 1000 units, consider adding to the antibiotic treatment the installation of a pleural drainage tube or pleural catheter depending on the size of the child, to prevent the process from progressing.

8.2 Fibrinopurulent phase

When there is macroscopic pus in the puncture, antibiotics along with a thick chest tube has been the traditional management, which has changed to thinner tubes or small diameter catheters that are easy to install and cause less pain to the patient, with a high success when said empyema is free [5]. Currently, most pediatric centers do not install traditional chest tubes but rather pig tail catheters for the treatment of non-septum empyema.

Once the septa are formed the pleural tube will evacuate fluid only from some locules of the septate empyema and will not be able to completely evacuate the fibrin clots that have formed especially in the pleuropulmonary spaces decubitus or destroy the partitions that have formed between the visceral and parietal pleura, for which video surgery is necessary for the removal of septa by debridement pleuropulmonary [44, 45].

If at this stage the installation of a thoracostomy tube fails to evacuate the purulent pleural fluid from the pleural space on the follow-up chest x-ray, it is surely the child already had septa formed. A surgeon must be consulted to ensure complete drainage through thoracoscopy, optionally with prior ultrasound.

8.3 Organization phase or fibrosis

When the final stage of fibrous sequela is reached, the antibiotics are not necessary and kinesiotherapy does not achieve lung re-expansion it is necessary to perform a formal pleuropulmonary decortication, which in the pediatric age is the exception, since it is generally possible to reverse the box fibrosis in several months [46]. For a stage III empyema in the organization phase, thoracostomy tube drainage alone will almost assuredly result in treatment failure and consideration for surgical intervention to definitively address the empyema may supplant the role of a thoracostomy tube.

9. Preoperative investigations and preparation

Dr. Richard W. Light has the merit of having differentiated from a physical-chemical point of view the pleural fluids in transudative effusion and exudative effusion more than 50 years ago [47, 48] and subsequently classified exudative effusion according to different criteria, being that of complicated parapneumonic effusions when the pH is equal to or less than 7.2, lactate dehydrogenase greater than 1000 units, glucose less than 40 mg/dL or less than 25% of the blood glucose level and the Gram stain or culture is positive [49]. Light's criteria are still accepted as the default reference test for separating transudates and pleural exudates after half a century [50].

Loculations or septations should have been shown with images. A consensus statement from the American College of Chest Physicians in 2000 noted an increase in interventions as the stage of effusion increased. Similarly, a pleural fluid pH of less than 7.1 has been found to result in a sixfold increase in the likelihood of surgical intervention based on retrospective data [51]. While these criteria document the pathophysiological progression of disease, the clinical relevance of the physicochemical analysis is not critical because the prognostic value is less important in the practice. Once pleural space debris causes symptoms and requires removal, drainage or surgery is required based on the nature of the debris.

10. Treatment

The classic treatment of the fibrinopurulent phase has been antibiotic therapy and pleural drainage with good success but with prolonged treatments and hospital stays.

In children in phase or stages exudative with small and same moderate-sized effusions were effectively managed without drainage (015). This suggests that intervention should also be based on symptoms and not just on the size of the effusion alone. The symptoms of intervention are tachypnea and increasing oxygen requirement [52].

When deciding to drain the fluid, options include single or multiple thoracentesis versus tube thoracostomy. It may be reasonable in an older child who tolerates the procedure with local anesthesia; probably would not be appropriate in younger children. The British Thoracic Society guidelines recommend a chest tube in cases where the first thoracentesis fails to adequately drain the effusion and thus avoid multiple attempts [53].

Almost all authors recommend the procedure with sedation in children according to local guidelines. The skin and soft tissues around the fifth intercostal space in the midaxillary line are asepticized according to each hospital's protocol and infiltrated with 1% lidocaine. A 12 Fr or larger chest tube can be used depending on the size of the child with the classic technique through a small incision or a pig tail catheter can be introduced using the Seldinger technique through a small incision and using dilators up to the desired number of catheters. Regarding appropriate chest tube sizing, no advantage has been confirmed with tubes larger than 14 Fr and on the other hand smaller caliber tubes are not hindered when used in spills. No differences have been found in pleural effusions in children treated with standard chest tubes compared to those treated with pigtail tubes. Image guidance is not considered necessary to guide the procedure in most patients but if you have the resources and expertise in handling the ultrasound transducer, you can use it. In some centers, the installation of the drain is performed under general anesthesia with tracheal intubation, especially in infants and preschoolers.

Once the tube or pig tail catheter is inserted, the fluid that is withdrawn is sent for physical-chemical study, Gram and bacteriological culture and the tube is attached to a – 20-centimeters H20 suction collection device and it is recommended to evaluate with a portable chest x-ray.

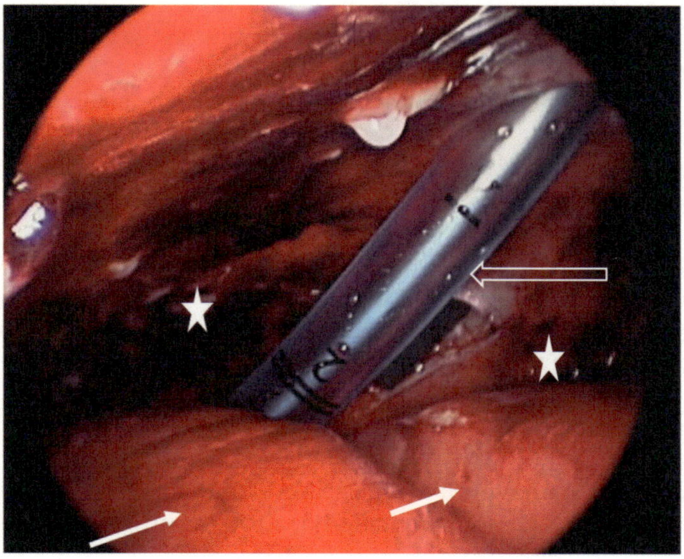

Figure 6.
Study of pneumonia that does not respond to treatment.

When a child with pneumonia does not respond to antibiotic treatment within 48 hours, a practical approach developed by the author is shown in **Figure 6**. A chest x-ray should always be indicated in this scenario. If there is no pleural effusion, the treating pediatrician continues the treatment of the pneumonia. If there is an effusion, the study must be complemented with ultrasound. If this shows septate fluid, a thoracoscopy is indicated (in some centers a fibrinolytic protocol is initiated as will be explained in detail later). If the pleural effusion is free on the ultrasound, the treatment is maintained and an evacuative pleurocentesis will be performed or a pleural drainage will be installed depending on the volume of the effusion and each case. The treatment is maintained, and the antibiotic can be adapted to the result of the culture and the sensitivity of the causative germ, if it is positive. The child will be monitored clinically and radiologically. If the drainage is partial and the child remains febrile with leukocytosis and elevated C-reactive protein 48 to 72 hours after the procedure, video-assisted thoracoscopy is proposed unless it is proven that the condition is due to necrotizing pneumonia.

When a child with free and small parapneumonic pleural effusion has an indication for pleurocentesis according to **Figures 5** and **6** is proposed. If the extracted fluid is purulent, a pleural drainage is installed and antibiotics are maintained according to the protocol of the local infections committee, which will be modified according to the results of the culture. If the pleurocentesis fluid is not macroscopically purulent and its laboratory study indicates that it is not complicated, antibiotics are continued. If it is considered that the pleural effusion is of limiting volume, the installation of a pleural drainage is added on a case-by-case basis. If the study of the fluid shows that it is complicated according to Light's criteria, a pleural drainage is installed regardless of the volume of the pleural effusion. All post-pleural drainage installation scenarios will be controlled clinically and radiologically.

11. Surgical treatment

With the formation of septa that trap the pleural fluid, the drainage tube becomes insufficient since it only manages to drain some locules, so the surgical release of the fibrin must be performed.

The goal of surgical treatment of pleural empyema in this phase is:

a. transform the multiloculated collection into a collection unique to achieve complete drainage of residual fluid.

b. debride fibrin as much as possible to control pleural infection and free the lung to expand and reestablish contact between the visceral pleura and the parietal pleura. In this way, the resolution of the infection is accelerated, achieves lung re-expansion and that antibiotic treatment be more effective. With minimally invasive techniques, obtain an excellent result, achieving post-operative with little pain, shorter hospital stays and good outcome esthetic [54, 55].

The critical consideration prior to embarking on thoracoscopic or open debridement for empyema is the status of the underlying parenchyma. Patients with persistent illness may have pulmonary necrosis as their source instead of pleural space disease. In this circumstance, an operation should be avoided in favor of patience.

The surgical technique described below corresponds to that used in our surgery service that we have performed for around 20 years. Some modifications have been the product of personal experience and exchange with American experts that we have visited and with some who have visited us.

For each of the following surgical techniques, the procedure is performed under general anesthesia with tracheal intubation facilitated by selective one-lung ventilation. The patient is placed in the lateral decubitus position with the affected side up and an axillary roll is placed. An attempt should be made to place the patient's iliac crest at the break point that all operating tables have. Subsequently, the table is angled at an angle greater than 180 degrees, which allows an expansion in the thorax that opens the intercostal spaces, facilitating the introduction and motility of either the trocars or the thoracoscopic instruments.

Initial incision and insertion of a 10 mm port being positioned in the area deemed advantageous for accessing the majority of disease after a review of the ultrasound images. Typically, this initial 10 mm port is best placed directly overlying the empyema. In infants and preschoolers, one of 5 mm trocar is preferred. The placement of the port in the fifth intercostal space at the mid-axillary line is also a good starting point. A low pressure (4 mmHg) and low flow (1 L/min) CO_2 pneumothorax facilitates lung collapse. A 10 or 5 mm angled telescope, depending on the first trocar is used to create a working space by freeing the virtual pleural space of septa or fibrinopus deposits from the lung to the chest wall with the end of the telescope.

As seen in the author's unpublished photographic series in **Figure 7**, the thoracoscopic view shows once the underlying lung has been adequately released and the 5 mm instrument has been introduced into the site where most of the fibrinopus must be released.

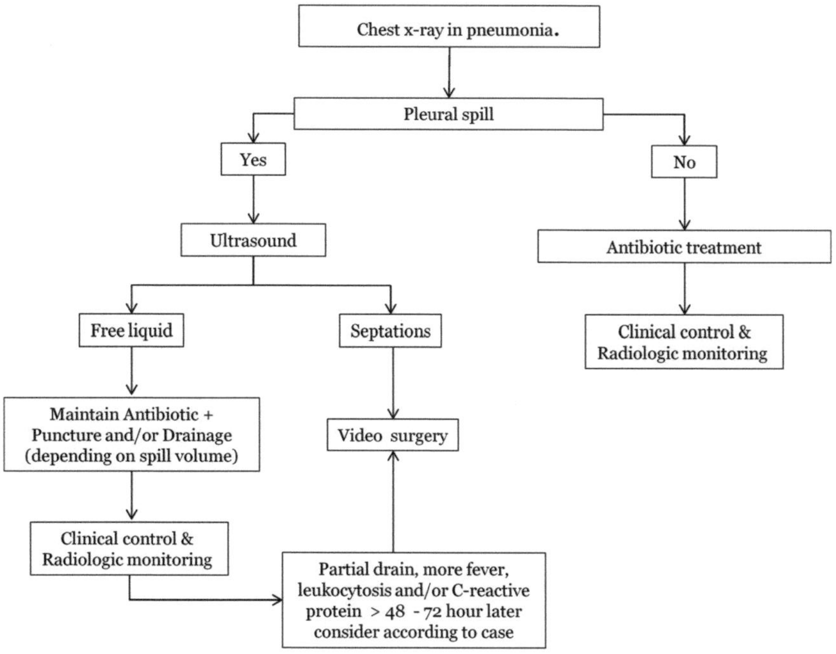

Figure 7.
The thoracoscopic view of a large amount of fibrinpus filling a fairly widened pleural space (asterisk) which do not initially allow visualization of the lung as is usual in advanced cases. The instrument (5 mm) being observed (arrow) will allow the lung to be released.

When two incisions are not enough a small third incision can be made for a second working port.

Other authors use a single trocar thoracoscopic operation with a conventional rigid scope with a working channel with good results in the treatment of pleural empyema in children [56].

Samples for physical-chemical study, Gram and bacteriological culture are routinely sent by attaching a Lukens trap to the suction device. In addition, fibrin is sent to histopathology, which can also help in trying to determine the microorganism.

For pleural debridement and peel are using a ring forceps or Yankauer suction devices. In adolescent children, alternatively, atraumatic grasping forceps from open surgery can also be used.

In **Figures 8–10** you can see how the thick fibrin pus shell adhered to the lung is carefully removed and the pleural cavity is released step by step. In photographs C and D, you can see that the underlying lung, at least at that level, is in good condition.

In order not to repeatedly remove fibrin fragments from the thorax with the instrument and reintroduce it again to continue debridement, it is useful and reduces surgical time to accumulate the fibrin in an accessible recess and at the end of debridement, remove or aspirate it at once.

In **Figure 11**, you can see that both pleurae have been freed from the fibrin pus. The surgical objective was obtained. Lung was re-expanded and pleura-to-pleura contact was achieved, which cannot be seen in the photography since we are still working with carbon dioxide pneumothorax that separates them.

Finally, in **Figure 12** you can see that the multiloculated collection has been transformed into a single collection and a soft and flexible chest drain is installed in the pleural space under direct vision.

To reduce the possibility of pneumothorax when the tube is removed, it should not be inserted directly from the skin to the pleura, so it is preferable to tunnel the

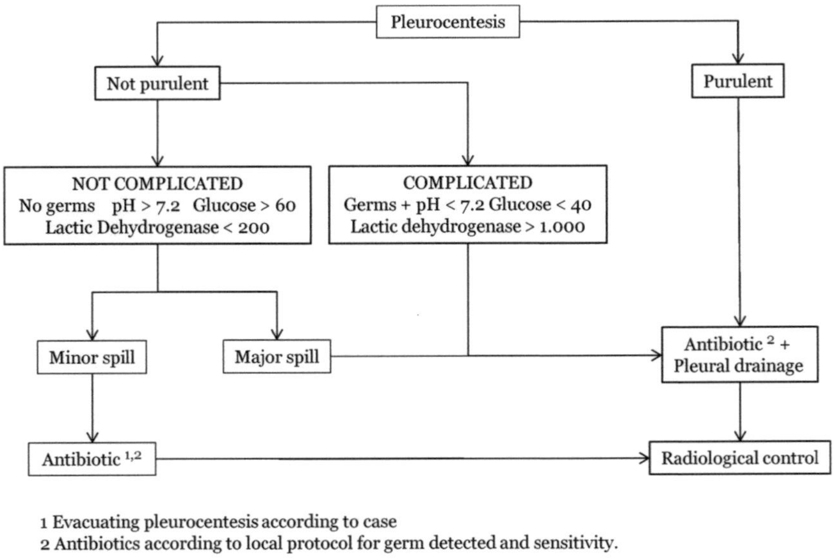

Figure 8.
Advancing the release, thick septa (asterisk) are observed on the upper edge that goes from the visceral to the parietal pleura. There are abundant deposits of fibrinopus adhered to the lung (unfilled arrow) and chest wall (single white arrow) and slowly space is opening (red arrow) up for better visualization.

DOI: http://dx.doi.org/10.5772/intechopen.114092

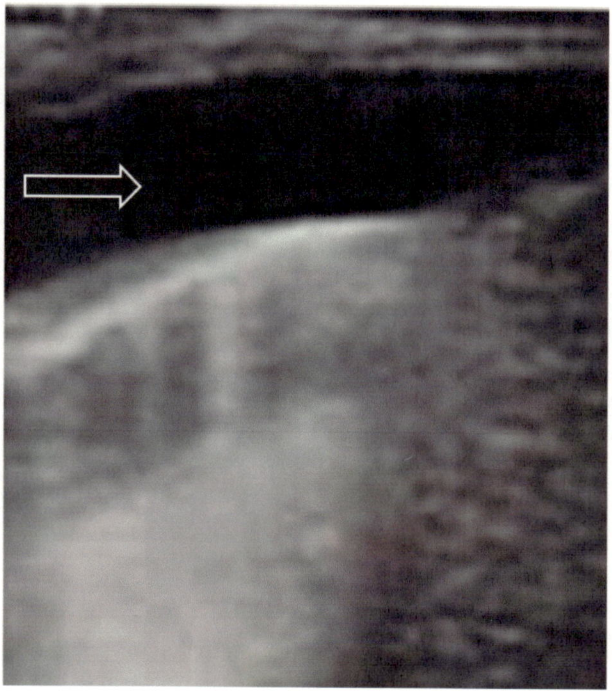

Figure 9.
The peel of fibrin pus over the lung has been partially released (Asterik). The lung is seen in good condition at that level (unfilled arrow).

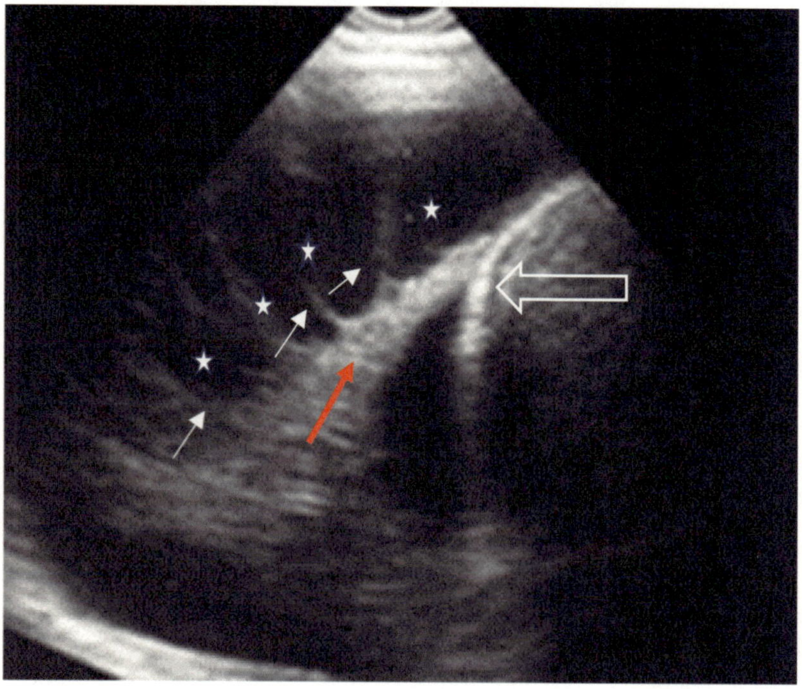

Figure 10.
Progressing in the release of the peel on the visceral pleural (black asterisk), reaching the edge of the lung lobe. At the level of the parietal pleura there is abundant fibrin pus (red asterisk). Lung (unfilled arrow).

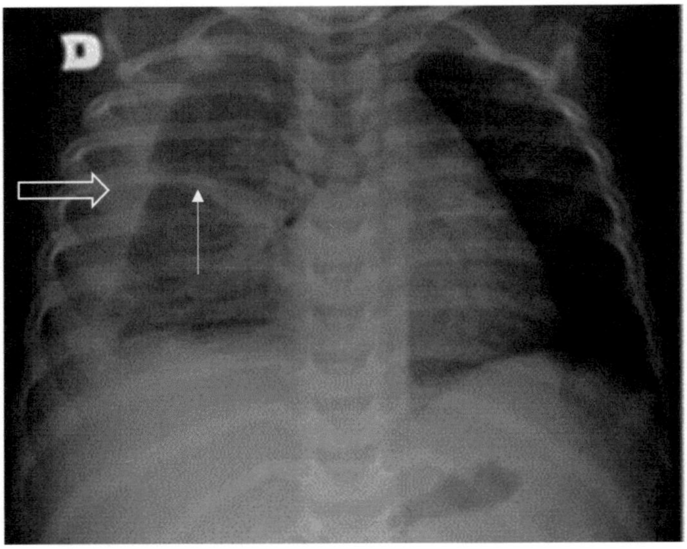

Figure 11.
Both the visceral (black asterisk) and parietal pleura (red arrow) have been freed from the fibrin pus. The surgical objective was obtained. Lung (unfilled arrow) was re-expanded and pleura-to-pleura contact was achieved, which cannot be seen in the photograph since we are still working with carbon dioxide pneumothorax that separates them.

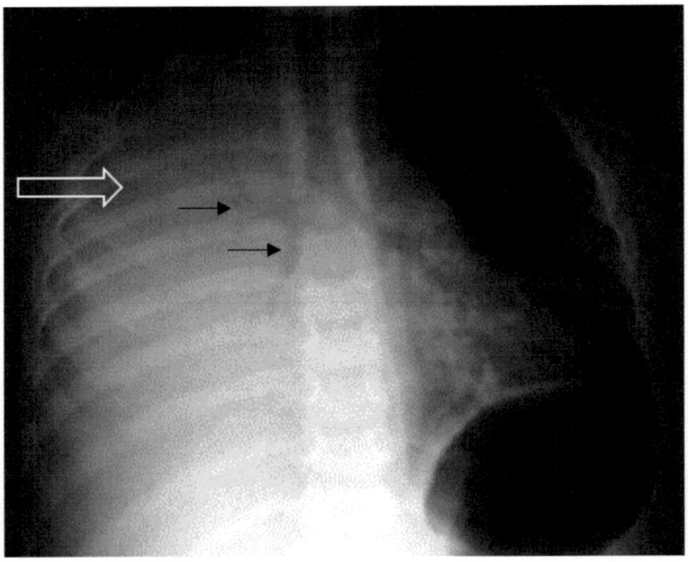

Figure 12.
The third surgical objective was achieved. Transform the multiloculated collection into a single collection (Asterik). Finally, a soft and flexible chest drain (Unfilled arrow) is installed in the pleural space under direct vision. Lung (single arrow).

drainage tube at the subcutaneous cellular level over the costal space in a cephalad direction to the site of the port where it enters the next pleural space.

Once the drainage tube is installed, it is fixed to the skin using a technique according to local protocol and the other incisions that were made are closed with absorbable suture and sterile dressings are applied to each one.

When video thoracoscopy equipment is not available, which is currently an exception, pleural debridement can be performed through a small thoracotomy. It is done under direct vision. Loculations of fibrin pus are released and eliminated. An appropriately sized chest drain is placed. The costal wall is closed in the usual manner. In the past, Raffensberger [57] recommended doing it with a two-centimeter resection of the rib, which is not accepted today.

12. Postoperative care

The chest drain is initially placed in a system with 20-centimeters water suction that is available from different commercial brands in different markets. If there are no air leaks or the output is not serious, you can switch to a bulb suction system (with springs) or to the classic underwater trap. A postoperative chest x-ray in the recovery room is necessary. Chest tube or catheter is removed once there is no evidence of air leakage and the drainage is less than 1 ml/kg/day in at least a 24-hour period, without the need for post-removal radiographs, unless otherwise indicated. After the drainage is removed, the incision is closed with absorbable suture or taking advantage of the suture with which, the tube had been fixed and sterile dressings are applied.

Pain should be treated according to local pain guidelines, initial non-invasive monitoring with oxygen supply as needed together with control of hemoglobin, hydrosaline and acid-base balance are necessary. Maintenance kinesiotherapy and antibiotics, according to crop must be modified.

There are no data from randomized controlled trials on the appropriate duration of the antibiotic or whether the duration should vary depending on the causative organism. Some continue intravenous antibiotics for 48 hours after the fever is gone. Others maintain it for a total of 7 to 10 days that the patient is afebrile. When switching to oral treatment, this should be continued for 2 to 3 weeks more [58]. The current consensus guidelines on empyema recommend antibiotics 10 days after the resolution of fever.

The child must remain hospitalized while connected to the drainage system and discharge is preferably based on clinical criteria: afebrile, no need for oxygen, the pain is controlled, good appetite with nutritional issues are optimized, good level of activity and general condition, rather than radiological criteria, since the radiograph chest lesions take between 4 to 8 weeks to clean after debridement and in some cases they still maintain some degree of residual pleural thickening until 12 to 24 weeks postoperatively. A follow-up visit and chest radiograph are recommended 3–4 weeks following discharge [58].

13. Complications

As treatments depend on the different phases or pathophysiological states of the pleural effusion, most children with parapneumonic effusion or empyema recover completely. In the majority of cases, both the lung parenchyma and the pleurae appear normal in the months after the event [59, 60].

Complications may be inherent to the pneumonia causing the effusion, of the empyema itself or its treatment like drainage tubes or catheter, thoracoscopy and vascular lines. We analyze them separately.

13.1 Complications inherent to the pneumonia

The lung can develop a serious complication such as necrotizing pneumonia. Cavitations may develop which can rupture and cause tension pneumothorax. A bronchopleural fistula may also occur in severe cases. These complications are rare, but if they occur, treatment is complex and recovery is prolonged [58]. Exceptionally, a perforation through the chest wall may occur, which is called empyema necessitans [61, 62].

13.2 Complications inherent to the pleural effusion and empyema

Arriving late to the treatment of exudate or empyema can cause its progression, reproduction of the process with greater complications or end in the last phase or stage of the process that traps the lung and causes a ventilatory restricted lung.

13.3 Complications inherent to the insertion of drainage tubes or catheters

Placing a thoracostomy tube or catheter is rare malposition, bleeding or wound infection at the exit site and persistent atelectasis. Also, can be associated with severe but very rare complications including damage to the lung, diaphragm, heart, liver or spleen, intercostal nerve or artery or vein injury. To avoid iatrogenesis and minimize complications, the use of ultrasound or another imaging modality such as fluoroscopy, may be used to guide placement of the thoracostomy tube or catheter [63, 64]. The increasingly common use of small tubes (pigtail catheters) has reduced installation complications and postoperative pain [65, 66].

During the insertion of drainage tubes or catheters, it is impossible to evaluate the presence of adhesions between the lung and the pleural surface when the patient has had previous pleuropulmonary processes. Knowing the child's previous medical/surgical history and the use of ultrasound before and during tube insertion minimize this potential complication [67].

13.4 Complications post insertion of the drainage tubes or catheter

Draining pleural fluid too quickly can occasionally cause pulmonary edema, known as "pulmonary reexpansion edema." It is recommended after draining the initial 10 ml/kg of pleural fluid to stop and clamp the tube for 1 hour to avoid sudden re-expansion. The tube is then unclamped and another 10 ml/kg of pleural fluid is allowed to drain if there is still any.

For adolescents, some experts suggest that drainage should be limited to 500 ml/hour with the previously mentioned 1-hour rest with the tube clamped. It is continued in the same way without exceeding a total of 1500 ml of pleural fluid [43, 68].

Reexpansion pulmonary edema usually arises after rapid reexpansion of a lung that has been collapsed for at least 3 days due to pneumothorax or effusion. An initial report reported that it was more likely after pneumothorax drainage; however, in later publications, it has been more associated with drainage of pleural effusions [69, 70].

If in the postoperative period the tube continuously bubbling, the position of the tube should be assessed since it may be partly out of the thorax with one of its drainage holes open to the atmosphere [58]. If the tube is *in situ* ok, the problem may also be caused by a bronchopleural fistula, especially in cases of necrotizing pneumonia, a complication that sometimes requires endoscopic or autologous blood therapy through drainage [71] and exceptionally with a surgical intervention.

Morbidity and mortality from thoracostomy tube or catheter placement are related to the experience and training of the clinician, the indication for placement and the circumstances under which the tube is placed: planned or urgency [72–75].

The complications of video thoracoscopy are those inherent to other thoracic surgeries and are beyond the objectives of the chapter, as are the complications of the venous and arterial lines used.

14. Fibrinolytics

The definitive management for empyema has traditionally been surgical debridement [76], which has historically been performed by video-assisted thoracic surgery (VATS) that has resulted in earlier and more complete resolution of empyema than chest tube drainage alone in both retrospective and prospective studies, translating shorter hospitalization with primary VATS. However, primary management of empyema with surgical debridement is changing and fibrinolysis has developed a more prominent role in empyema management.

The British Thoracic Society recommended years ago fibrinolytic therapy as a medical option for patients in whom fluid pleural is thick or septate as a reasonable alternative to videothoracoscopy for children with parapneumonic effusion septum who are hospitalized in institutions that lack from a pediatric surgeon trained in videothoracoscopy, based on the fact that there are no differences in the clinical results [58] and another author has very similar results with both methods except for the lower cost with the use of fibrinolytics [77].

Three prospective, randomized trials compared fibrinolysis with VATS in the treatment of pleural empyema in children more than 10 years ago. They were carried out in three countries. Spain [78], the United Kingdom [79] and the United States [80] in 103, 60 and 36 patients respectively. All three studies compared the installation of fibrinolytic agents for 3 days to VATS as the initial therapy for empyema. The first fibrinolytic dose in both studies was given upon diagnosis and/or chest tube placement. The Spanish study used urokinase every 12 hours for 3 days while the other two studies used every 24-hour to complete the three-dose. The results were concordant, with all the studies documenting no difference in the duration of hospitalization, the primary outcome in all the trials. The failure rate for fibrinolysis was 10% in the Spanish study and 16.6% in the other two studies. These failure rates were similar to previous studies investigating the utility of fibrinolysis, so that fibrinolysis is an effective first-line therapy.

Fibrinolysis is performed by mixing 4 mg of tissue plasminogen activator (tPA) = Alteplase ® in 40 mL of normal saline which is injected directly into the tube, which is then clapped for 1 hour. After the dwell time, the tube returns to continuous suction. Two additional doses are then administered at 24-hour intervals using the same technique. If, after three doses, the patient has not clinically improved, another ultrasound is performed to evaluate for intrapleural disease. Minimally invasive pleural debridement is considered eventually if the tissue plasminogen activator (tPA) has failed to eradicate the pleural space of fibrinopurulent material [81].

An interesting retrospective single-center observational study of 97 children hospitalized in Belgium, with a diagnosis of parapneumonic pleural effusion during a 15-year period, indicates that corticosteroids may be a part of the therapeutic armamentarium for children with parapneumonic effusion when conventional nonsurgical management fails, especially when the fever does not subside, as an anti-inflammatory therapy [82].

In our country, the high cost of urokinase has not allowed its use to be introduced, except in isolated cases, so there is not enough experience. In particular, the use of Alteplase ® is being initiated in our hospital, so we do not have objective results.

Keypoints

- An early clinical diagnosis of parapneumonic effusions is important.

- The most common symptoms of empyema are fever, cough, malaise, anorexia, chest pain, dyspnea or lack of response within 48 hours of appropriate therapy for pneumonia.

- Children with the described symptoms should be evaluated with chest x-ray.

- If the radiological effusion is greater than 1 cm in lateral decubitus radiography or a quarter of the hemithorax in the upright position, an ultrasound should be continued, which is the image indicated to confirm the presence of fluid in the pleural space and evaluate loculations and septa.

- If the effusion is free, a diagnostic pleurocentesis should be added if the liquid is scarce.

- Depending on the type and amount of spillage, a tube or catheter pleural should be placed.

- If the spill reproduces or is blocked, the best recommendation is video-assisted thoracoscopy to perform a pleuropulmonary debridement that improves the child in minor time and with fewer sequelae.

- If the center has experience and practice in fibrinolytic therapies, an initial attempt is a good decision based on controlled trials that show no significant difference in several important outcome variables.

- The author declares that he has no conflicts of interest in relation to this article.

Author details

Iván Alcoholado Boye
University of Chile, Chile

*Address all correspondence to: ialcoholado@alemana.cl

References

[1] Tuomanen EI, Austrian R, Masure HR. Pathogenesis of pneumococcal infection. The New England Journal of Medicine. 1995;**332**:1280-1284

[2] Bryan RE, Salomon CJ. Pleural Empyema. Clinical Infectious Diseases. 1996;**22**:747-764

[3] Ren Y, Okazaki T, Ngamsnae P, Hashimoto H, Ikeda R, Honkura Y, et al. Anatomy and function of the lymphatic vessels in the parietal pleura and their plasticity under inflammation in mice. Microvascular Research. 2023;**148**:104546. DOI: 10.1016

[4] Osório C, Carvalho L. Ana Marta Pereira, Mário Nora, Marta Guimarães Acute. Pericarditis hiding an esophageal perforation. Cureus. 2022;**14**(12):e32608. DOI: 10.7759

[5] Zineb J, Moboula C, Meryem N, Abdallah F, Kamilia C, Souhail B. *Staphylococcus aureus* bacteremia with a mediastinal abscess in a 9-month-old infant: A case report and literature review. The Pan African Medical Journal. 2023;**44**:173. DOI: 10.11604

[6] Byington CL, Spencer LY, Johnson TA, et al. An epidemiological investigation of a sustained high rate of pediatric parapneumonic empyema: Risk factors and microbiological associations. Clinical Infectious Diseases. 2002;**34**:434

[7] Bradley JS, Byington CL, Shah SS, et al. The management of community-acquired pneumonia in infants and children older than 3 months of age: Clinical practice guidelines by the Pediatric Infectious Diseases Society and the Infectious Diseases Society of America. Clinical Infectious Diseases. 2011;**53**:e25-e76

[8] Hoff SJ, Neblett WW, Edwards KM, et al. Parapneumonic empyema in children: Decortication hastens recovery in patients with severe pleural infections. The Pediatric Infectious Disease Journal. 1991;**10**:194

[9] Hardie W, Bokulic R, Garcia VF, et al. Pneumococcal pleural empyemas in children. Clinical Infectious Diseases. 1996;**22**:1057

[10] Lewis KT, Bukstein DA. Parapneumonic empyema in children: Diagnosis and management. American Family Physician. 1992;**46**:1443

[11] Ampofo K, Herbener A, Blaschke AJ, et al. Association of 2009 pandemic influenza a (H1N1) infection and increased hospitalization with parapneumonic empyema in children in Utah. The Pediatric Infectious Disease Journal. 2010;**29**:905

[12] Golladay ES, Wagner CW. Management of empyema in children. American Journal of Surgery. 1989;**158**:618

[13] Brook I. Microbiology of empyema in children and adolescents. Pediatrics. 1990;**85**:722

[14] St L, Tancredi DJ. Empyema hospitalizations increased in US children despite pneumococcal conjugate vaccine. Pediatrics. 2010;**125**:26-33

[15] Chonmaitree T, Powell KR. Parapneumonic pleural effusion and empyema in children. Review of a 19-year experience, 1962-1980. Clinical Pediatrics (Phila). 1983;**22**:414

[16] Freitas M, Castelo A, Petty G, Gomes CE, Carvalho E. Viridans

streptococci causing community acquired pneumonia. Archives of Disease in Childhood. 2006;**91**:779-780

[17] Givan DC, Eigen H. Common pleural effusions in children. Clinics in Chest Medicine. 1998;**19**:363-371

[18] Moses AE, Ziv A, Harari M, Rahav G, Shapiro M, Englehard D. Increased incidence and severity of streptococcus pyogenes bacteremia in young children. The Pediatric Infectious Disease Journal. 1995;**14**:767-770

[19] Arancibia MF, Vega-Briceño LE, Pizarro ME, Pulgar D, Holmgren NL, Bertrand P, et al. Empiema y efusión pleural en niños. Revista Chilena de Infectología. 2007;**24**(6):454-461ren. Pediatr Infect Dis J 1995; 14:767-770

[20] Chan K-PF, Ma T-F, Sridhar S, Lam DC-L, Ip MS-M, Ho P-L. Changes in etiology and clinical outcomes of pleural empyema during the COVID-19 pandemic. Microorganisms. 2023;**11**(2):303. DOI: 10.3390

[21] Kaddour M, Simeonovic M, Osowicki J, McNab S, Satzke C, Robertson C, et al. COVID-19 and complicated bacterial pneumonia in children. ERJ Open Research. 2021;**7**(1):00884-02020. DOI: 10.1183/23120541

[22] van Kempen EB, Bruijning-Verhagen PCJ, Borensztajn D, Vermont CL, Quaak MSW, Janson J-A, et al. Increase in invasive group a streptococcal infections in children in the Netherlands, a survey among 7 hospitals in 2022. The Pediatric Infectious Disease Journal. 2023;**42**(4):e122-e124

[23] Michelson KA, Dart AH, Bachur RG, Mahajan P, Finkelstein JA. Measuring complications of serious pediatric emergencies using ICD-10. Health Services Research. 2021;**56**(2):225-234. DOI: 10.1111/1475-6773.13615

[24] Ghaffar S, Khan IA, Asif S, Rahman ZU. Empyema thoracis: Management outcome. Journal of Ayub Medical College, Abbottabad. 2010;**22**(3):12-14

[25] Ahn HY, Cho JS, Kim YD, Hoseok I, Song S, Eom JS, et al. Factors affecting postoperative lung expansion in patients with pyogenic empyema. The Thoracic and Cardiovascular Surgeon. 2018;**66**(8):697-700

[26] Wiese AD, Griffin MR, Zhu Y, et al. Changes in empyema among U.S. children in the pneumococcal conjugate vaccine era. Vaccine. 2016;**34**:6243

[27] Madhi F, Levy C, Morin L, et al. Change in bacterial causes of community-acquired parapneumonic effusion and pleural empyema in children 6 years after 13-valent pneumococcal conjugate vaccine implementation. Journal of the Pediatric Infectious Diseases Society. 2019;**8**:474

[28] de Miguel S, Pérez-Abeledo M, Ramos B, García L, Arce A, Martínez-Arce R, et al. Distribution of multidrug-resistant invasive serotypes of *Streptococcus pneumoniae* during the period 2007-2021 in Madrid, Spain. Antibiotics (Basel). 2023;**12**(2):342. DOI: 10.3390/antibiotics12020342

[29] Angurana SK, Kumar R, Singh M, Verma S, Samujh R, Singhi S. Pediatric empyema thoracis: What has changed over a decade? Journal of Tropical Pediatrics. 2019;**65**(3):231-239. North India

[30] Zhang X, Zhang H. Microbiological characteristics and outcomes of children with pleural empyema admitted to a tertiary hospital in Southeast China,

2009-2018. The Turkish Journal of Pediatrics. 2021;**63**(6):994-1003

[31] Rodgers BM, McGahren ED. Mediastinum and pleura. In: Oldham KT, Colombani PM, Foglia RP, Skinner MA, editors. Principles and Practice of Pediatric Surgery. Philadelphia: Lippincott Williams & Wilkins; 2005. p. 929

[32] Thys JP, Vanderhoeft P, Herchuelz A, Bergmann P, Yourassowsky E. Penetration of aminoglycosides in uninfected pleural exudates and in pleural empyemas. Chest. 1988;**93**(3):530-532

[33] Teixeira LR, Sasse SA, Villarino MA, Nguyen T, Mulligan ME, Light RW. Antibiotic levels in empyemic pleural fluid. Chest. 2000;**117**(6):1734-1739

[34] Harris M, Clark J, Coote N, Fletcher P, McKean M, Thomson A. British Thoracic Society standards of care committee. British Thoracic Society guidelines for the management of community acquired pneumonia in children: Update 2011. Thorax. 2011;**66**(Suppl 2):ii1-i23

[35] Carter E, Waldhausen J, Zhang W, et al. Management of children with empyema: Pleural drainage is not always necessary. Pediatric Pulmonology. 2010;**45**:475-480

[36] Himelman RB, Callen PW. The prognostic value of loculations in parapneumonic pleural effusions. Chest. 1986;**90**:852-856

[37] Buchberger B, Scholl K, Krabbe L, Spiller L, Lux B. Radiation exposure by medical X-ray applications. German Medical Science. 2022;**20**:Doc06. DOI: 10.3205/000308

[38] Baysson H, Journy N, Roué T, Ducou-Lepointe H, Etard C, Bernier M-O. Exposure to CT scans in childhood and long-term cancer risk: A review of epidemiological studies. Bulletin du Cancer. 2016;**103**(2):190-198

[39] Pierrepoint MJ, Evans A, Morris SJ, Harrison SK, Doull IJ. Pigtail catheter drain in the treatment of empyema thoracis. Archives of Disease in Childhood. 2002;**87**:331-332

[40] Ramnath RR. Pediatris. 1998;**101**:68-71

[41] Donnelly LF, Klosterman LA. CT appearance of parapneumonic effusions in children: Findings are not specific for empyema. AJR. American Journal of Roentgenology. 1997;**169**:179-182

[42] Buckingham SC, King MD, Miller ML. Incidence and etiologies of complicated parapneumonic effusions in children, 1996 to 2001. The Pediatric Infectious Disease Journal. 2003;**22**:499-504

[43] Trapnell DH, Thurston JG. Unilateral pulmonary oedema after pleural aspiration. Lancet. 1970;**1**:1367-1369

[44] Panitch HB, Papastamelos C, Schidlow DV. Abnormalities of the pleural space. In: Taussig LM, Landau LI, editors. Pediatric Respiratory Medicine. St. Louis: Mosby; 1999. p. 1184

[45] Moran JF. Surgical management of pleural space infections. Seminars in Respiratory Infections. 1988;**3**:383-394

[46] Kennedy AS, Agness M, Bailey L, White JJ. Decortication for childhood empyema. The primary provider's peccadillo. Archives of Surgery. 1991;**126**:1287-1291

[47] Light RW, Girard WM, Jenkinson SG, George RB. Parapneumonic effusions. The American Journal of Medicine. 1980;**69**:507-512

[48] Light RW, Macgregor MI, Luchsinger PC, Ball WC Jr. Pleural effusions: The diagnostic separation of transudates and exudates. Annals of Internal Medicine. 1972;**77**:507-513

[49] Light RW. A new classification of parapneumonic effusions and empyema. Chest. 1995;**108**:299-301

[50] Porcel JM, Light RW. Pleural fluid analysis: Are light's criteria still relevant after half a century? Clinics in Chest Medicine. 2021;**42**(4):599-609

[51] Wong KS, Lin TY, Huang YC, et al. Scoring system for empyema thoracis and help in management. Indian Journal of Pediatrics. 2005;**72**:1025-1028

[52] Soares P, Barreira J, Pissarra S, et al. Pediatric parapneumonic pleural effusions: Experience in a university central hospital. Revista Portuguesa de Pneumologia. 2009;**15**:241-259

[53] Maskell N. British Thoracic Society pleural disease guideline group. British Thoracic Society pleural disease guidelines—2010 update. Thorax. 2010;**65**:667-669

[54] Jaffé A, Balfour-Lynn IM. Management of empyema in children. Pediatric Pulmonology. 2005;**40**:148-156

[55] Schultz KD, Fan LL, Pinsky J, Ochoa L, Smith EO, Kaplan SL, et al. The changing face of pleural empyemas in children: Epidemiology and management. Pediatrics. 2004;**113**:1735-1740

[56] Do Manh H, Thanh QN, Thanh LN, Van LN. Single trocar thoracoscopic surgery for pleural empyema in children. Journal of Laparoendoscopic & Advanced Surgical Techniques. Part A. 2023;**33**(7):707-712

[57] Raffensperger JG, editor. Swenson*s Pediatric Surgery. 5th ed. Conn: Appleton & Lange Norwalk; 1990

[58] Balfour-Lynn IM, Abrahamson E, Cohen G, Hartley J, King S, Parikh D, et al. Paediatric pleural diseases subcommittee of the BTS standards of care committee. BTS guidelines for the management of pleural infection in children. Thorax. 2005;**60**(Suppl. 1):i1-i21

[59] Cohen E, Mahant S, Dell SD, et al. The long-term outcomes of pediatric pleural empyema: A prospective study. Archives of Pediatrics & Adolescent Medicine. 2012;**166**:999

[60] Honkinen M, Lahti E, Svedström E, et al. Long-term recovery after parapneumonic empyema in children. Pediatric Pulmonology. 2014;**49**:1020

[61] White-Dzuro CG, Assi PE, Thomas HC, Thayer WP. Unusual presentation of empyema necessitans: Case report and review of the literature. General Thoracic and Cardiovascular Surgery. 2021;**69**(6):1026-1030

[62] Goussard P, Gie R, Janson J, Andronikou S. Empyema necessitans in a six-month-old girl. Paediatrics and International Child Health. 2019;**39**(3):224-226

[63] Menegozzo CAM, Utiyama EM. Steering the wheel towards the standard of care: Proposal of a step-by-step ultrasound-guided emergency chest tube drainage and literature review. International Journal of Surgery. 2018;**56**:315

[64] Hunnam GR, Flower CD. Radiologically-guided percutaneous catheter drainage of empyemas. Clinical Radiology. 1988;**39**:121

[65] Mei F, Rota M, Bonifazi M, Zuccatosta L, Porcarelli FM, Sediari M, et al. Efficacy of small versus large-bore chest drain in pleural infection: A systematic review and meta-analysis. Respiration. 2023;**102**(3):247-256

[66] Hamad A-MM, Alfeky SE. Small-bore catheter is more than an alternative to the ordinary chest tube for pleural drainage. Lung India. 2021;**38**(1):31-35

[67] Rafiq S, Dar MA, Nazir I, Shaffi F, Shaheen F, Kuchay IA. Image-guided catheter drainage in loculated pleural space collections, effectiveness, and complications. Lung India. 2020;**37**(4):316-322

[68] Laws D, Neville E, Duffy J. Pleural diseases group, standards of care committee, British Thoracic Society. BTS guidelines for the insertion of a chest drain. Thorax. 2003;**58 Suppl 2**:ii53

[69] Feller-Kopman D, Berkowitz D, Boiselle P, Ernst A. Large-volume thoracentesis and the risk of reexpansion pulmonary edema. The Annals of Thoracic Surgery. 2007;**84**:1656

[70] Adegboye VO, Falade A, Osinusi K, Obajimi MO. Reexpansion pulmonary oedema as a complication of pleural drainage. The Nigerian Postgraduate Medical Journal. 2002;**9**:214

[71] Lillegard JB, Kennedy RD, Ishitani MB, Zarroug AE, Feltis B. Autologous blood patch for persistent air leak in children. Journal of Pediatric Surgery. 2013;**48**:1862-1866

[72] Kwiatt M, Tarbox A, Seamon MJ, et al. Thoracostomy tubes: A comprehensive review of complications and related topics. International Journal of Critical Illness and Injury Science. 2014;**4**:143

[73] Ball CG, Lord J, Laupland KB, et al. Chest tube complications: How well are we training our residents? Canadian Journal of Surgery. 2007;**50**:450

[74] Collop NA, Kim S, Sahn SA. Analysis of tube thoracostomy performed by pulmonologists at a teaching hospital. Chest. 1997;**112**:709

[75] Wen KZ, Brereton CJ, Douglas EM, Samuel SRN, Jones AC. Pleural procedures: An audit of practice and complications in a regional Australian teaching hospital. Internal Medicine Journal. Jan 2024;**54**(1):172-177. DOI: 10.1111/imj.16147

[76] Pogorelić Z, Bjelanović D, Gudelj R, Jukić M, Petrić J, Furlan D. Video-assisted thoracic surgery in early stage of pediatric pleural empyema improves outcome. The Thoracic and Cardiovascular Surgeon. 2021;**69**(5):475-480

[77] Sonnappa S, Cohen G, Owens CM, van Doorn C, Cairns J, Stanojevic S, et al. Comparison of urokinase and video-assisted thoracoscopic surgery for treatment of childhood empyema. American Journal of Respiratory and Critical Care Medicine. 2006;**174**:221-227

[78] Marhuenda C, Barceló C, Fuentes I, et al. Urokinase versus VATS for treatment of empyema: A randomized multicenter clinical trial. Pediatrics. 2014;**134**(5):e1301-e1307

[79] Singh M, Mathew JL, Chandra S, et al. Randomized controlled trial of intrapleural streptokinase in empyema thoracis in children. Acta Paediatrica. 2004;**93**(11):1443-1445

[80] St Peter SD, Tsao K, Spilde TL, et al. Thoracoscopic decortication vs tube thoracostomy with fibrinolysis for

empyema in children: A prospective, randomized trial. Journal of Pediatric Surgery. 2009;**44**(1):106-111

[81] BTS Pleural Guideline Development Group. British Thoracic Society guideline for pleural disease. Thorax. 2023;**78**(Suppl 3):s1-s42. DOI: 10.1136/thorax-2022-219784

[82] Thimmesch M, Mulder A, Lebrun F, Piérart F, Genin C, Loeckx I, et al. Management of parapneumonic pleural effusion in children: Is there a role for corticosteroids when conventional nonsurgical management fails? A single-center 15-year experience. Pediatric Pulmonology. 2022;**57**(1):245-252

Section 2

Tuberculosis

Chapter 3

Pleural Tuberculosis

Yagnang Vyas

Abstract

Pleural tuberculosis (TB) is the second most common extra-pulmonary form of TB, following tuberculous lymphadenitis. Pleural TB is most likely to occur due to the rupture of a subpleural caseous focus within the lung or, sometimes, due to the spread of infection from a lymph node into the pleural space. In pleural TB, it has been found that the delayed type of hypersensitivity (DTH) is responsible for the development of pleural effusion. Clinical manifestations mainly include pleuritic chest pain, nonproductive cough, anorexia, weight loss, night sweats, and in severe cases, dyspnea. Manifestations of pleural TB among HIV individuals depend on the CD4 count. A chest radiograph is the initial mode of investigation and is confirmed by USG thorax. Pleural fluid analysis helps in diagnosing and ruling out other causes of pleural TB. Levels of ADA and interferon gamma are helpful in establishing the diagnosis of pleural TB. Pleural biopsy culture, in combination with histopathological and molecular methods, can diagnose up to 95% of pleural TB. Anti-tuberculous drugs are the mainstay of therapy and the duration of treatment is 6 months. The role of corticosteroids is limited to certain situations only. Residual pleural fibrosis is the most common complication, while TB empyema is a severe form of complication.

Keywords: pleural tuberculosis, pleural effusion, pleural TB, tuberculosis, *Mycobacterium tuberculosis*

1. Introduction

Pleural tuberculosis (TB) is the second most common extra-pulmonary form of TB, following tuberculous lymphadenitis. The incidence of pleural TB varies from 3 to 5% of tuberculous patients in non-endemic areas and can reach up to 30% in endemic areas [1, 2]. In countries like India, where there is a high burden of TB cases, the incidence of pleural TB varies from 30 to 80% of all pleural effusions and complicates 31% of Pleural TB [3]. The frequency of pleural TB depends on the prevalence of TB and HIV in a specific population. One should consider the diagnosis of TB in the presence of exudative pleural effusion.

2. Pathogenesis

Pleural TB is caused by *Mycobacterium tuberculosis* (Mtb) or nontuberculous mycobacteria (NTM). The majority of cases are associated with Mtb infection, but it may rarely be caused by NTM.

Pleural TB is most likely to occur due to the rupture of a subpleural caseous focus within the lung [4, 5], or sometimes due to the spread of infection from lymph nodes into the pleural space. This mechanism is more commonly observed in post-primary or secondary tuberculosis. Other postulated mechanisms include (1) hematogenous spread, as seen in the case of primary tuberculosis; (2) direct involvement of the pleura, which can occur in immunocompromised patients such as those with HIV/AIDS; and (3) spread from surrounding organ TB foci, such as TB spine, TB chest wall, or TB osteitis of the rib; (4) The involvement of peripheral interstitial lymphatics in TB may be responsible for the development of pleural effusion [6].

The development of pleural effusion depends on the rate of fluid formation and absorption. The formation of fluid depends on hydrostatic and oncotic pressure within the parietal and visceral pleura, as well as intrapleural pressure. Movement is governed by Starling's law. Change in this equation results in the accumulation of fluid from either parietal or visceral pleural capillaries. Interstitial fluid typically originates from high pressure or high permeability pulmonary edema. Other less common sources of pleural fluid include intrathoracic lymphatic or blood vessels and the peritoneal cavity. Fluid is reabsorbed by pleural lymphatics primarily in the parietal pleura and capillaries of the visceral pleura.

In pleural TB, it has been found that the delayed type of hypersensitivity (DTH) is responsible for the development of pleural effusion. Direct infection in the pleural space is rarely observed. The patient developed a reaction to Mtb protein, which reached the pleural space through the mechanism mentioned above, resulting in an inflammatory reaction due to interaction with T-lymphocytes. An increase in vascular permeability leads to the extravasation of protein-rich fluid. Additionally, a high concentration of protein within the pleural space stimulates the accumulation of fluid [7]. It also found that the lymphatic system stomas present in the parietal pleura are obstructed due to inflammation, ultimately resulting in a reduced rate of pleural fluid clearance [8].

The immunological reaction in response to Mtb protein within the pleural space is no different from that seen in the case of pulmonary TB. Initially, neutrophils play an important role, followed by macrophages and lymphocytes. Ultimately, a granuloma is formed, which can be visible on the parietal and visceral pleura during thoracoscopy.

3. Clinical manifestations

Pleural tuberculosis is typically an acute illness and is commonly observed in younger populations as part of primary tuberculosis. In the older population, it occurs as a part of post-primary tuberculosis. Diabetes mellitus (DM), chronic alcoholism, immunocompromised conditions such as HIV/AIDS, malignancy, post-organ transplant, immunosuppressive therapy, chronic kidney disease, etc., are risk factors for pleural TB.

The presentation of pleural tuberculosis varies in duration, ranging from a few days to several weeks or even months. Patients usually experience a dry cough and pleuritic chest pain, which worsens with coughing or sudden movement and is sometimes relieved by lying on the same side. When a presentation is acute, the predominant symptom is chest pain. In a chronic course, symptoms are milder in nature. Fever is present and is usually low-grade. Other symptoms are nonspecific, such as anorexia, night sweats, fatigue, and weight loss [1, 4, 8]. Sometimes, patients may remain completely asymptomatic [1].

Physical examination findings in such patients are usually nonspecific. Mediastinal shift of the trachea to the opposite side, fullness of the intercostal space, and reduced tactile vocal fremitus may be observed. In percussion, a subtympanic note is present at the level of pleural effusion and a stony dullness note is present in the case of large or massive pleural effusion. The obliteration of Traube's sign refers to the loss of the tympanic note in the left lower lung in the mid-axillary line, which is replaced by a dull note due to pleural effusion. The Ellis S-shaped curve sign is characterized by the highest dull note being present in the mid-axillary line and the lowest at the spine, assuming the shape of an S. This sign is observed in cases of moderate-sized effusion. Grocco's triangle sign is observed in cases of moderate to large effusion, where an area of dullness or decreased resonance is detected contralateral to the effusion at the lower side. It occurs due to the shift of the posterior mediastinum. During auscultation, air entry may be reduced or absent on the side with effusion. One can hear pleural friction rub during an acute presentation. The Aegophony sign is present, and vocal resonance is reduced in pleural effusion. All of the above examination findings are nonspecific and may be present in other causes of pleural effusion.

3.1 In HIV-positive individuals

In certain geographic areas, the incidence of TB and pleural TB has increased, which is attributed to the rise in HIV infections. Initially, it was thought that pleural TB tends to occur in the initial phase of HIV infection. However, it was found that it is more common among patients with a CD4 count greater than 200 cells per mL-1 [9]. Manifestations of pleural TB among HIV individuals depend on the CD4 count. In such individuals, in addition to delayed-type hypersensitivity (DTH), the persistence of Mtb within the pleural space due to immune system failure is proposed as a factor in the development of pleural TB [10]. Clinical features in HIV-positive individuals are similar to those in HIV-negative individuals, but patients may present with atypical, longer duration of symptoms and more severe complications.

4. Investigations

Once a patient is suspected to have pleural TB based on clinical presentation and physical examination, the next most appropriate step is to perform imaging to confirm the presence of pleural effusion.

4.1 Radiology

4.1.1 Chest x-ray

A chest radiograph is the most cost-effective and widely available method for further evaluating suspected pleural TB. Pleural effusion in tuberculosis is usually unilateral [11] and is present in 90% of cases, but bilateral involvement may also occur (see **Figures 1** and 2).

The chest x-ray in **Figure 1** shows unilateral pleural effusion, which is more commonly found on the right side. In **Figure 2**, the chest x-ray shows bilateral pleural effusion, which is present in about 10% of cases.

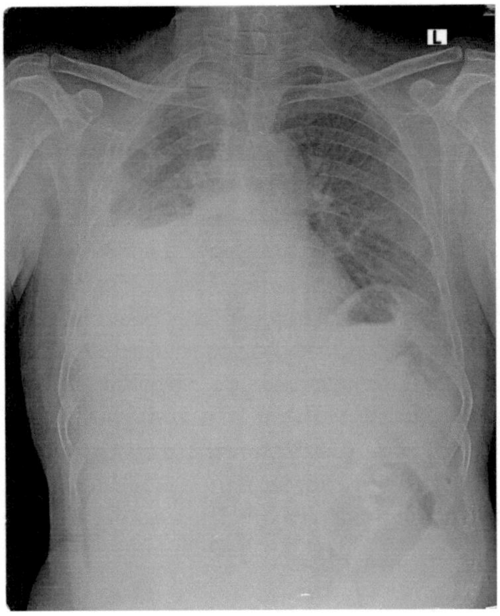

Figure 1.
Right side unilateral pleural effusion.

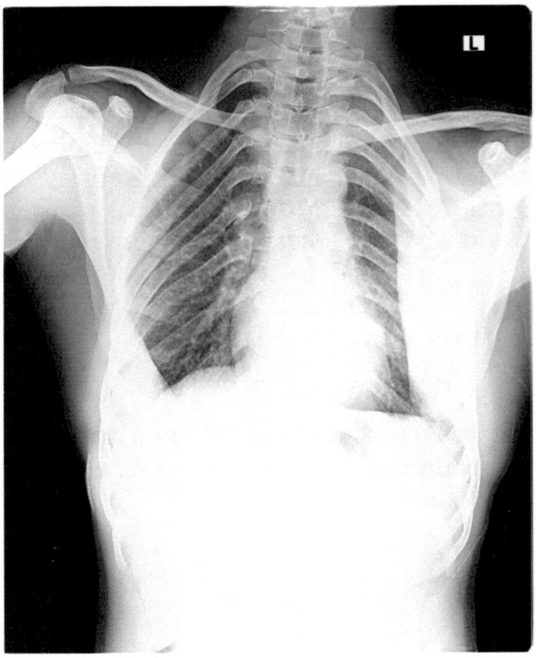

Figure 2.
Bilateral pleural effusion.

The amount of pleural effusion in tuberculosis varies from minimal to mild and can be large or even massive, leading to severe breathlessness in some patients. The amount of fluid in pleural TB commonly varies from mild to moderate [12].

In **Figure 3**, the chest x-ray suggests a massive pleural effusion with a shift of the mediastinum to the opposite side. In **Figure 4**, the chest x-ray shows a typical type of pleural TB. Sometimes, patients may present with loculated pleural effusion, as seen in **Figure 5**.

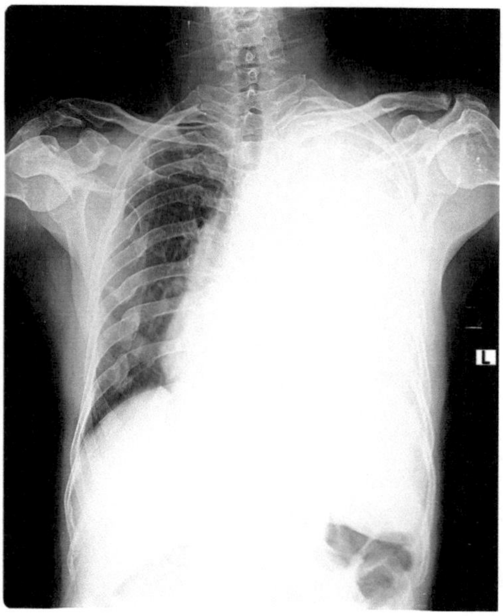

Figure 3.
Massive pleural effusion.

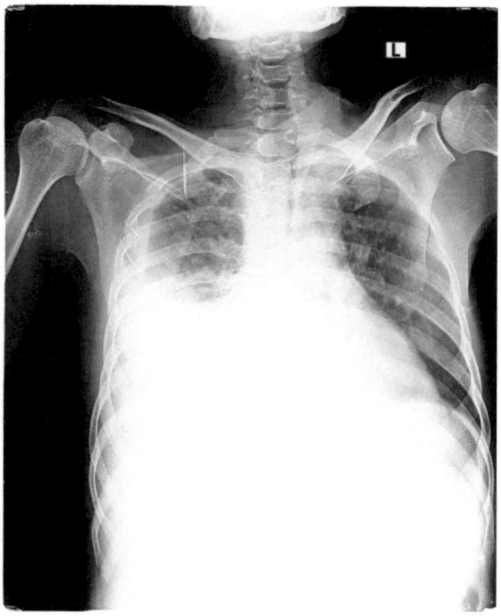

Figure 4.
Mild to moderate pleural effusion.

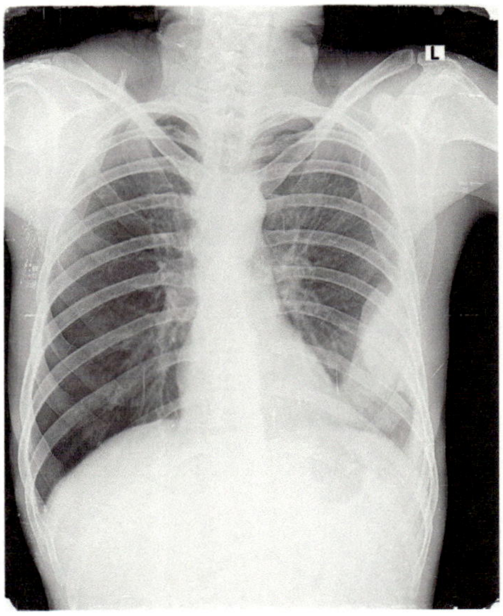

Figure 5.
Left Loculated pleural effusion.

4.1.2 Ultrasonography

Ultrasonography (USG) of the thorax is the most accurate method for confirming the presence and quantifying pleural fluid. It can more accurately detect effusion than a chest radiograph, without any exposure to radiation (**Figure 6**).

On ultrasonography (USG), the most common findings in pleural TB are homogeneously echogenic, septated, or complex. The presence of echogenic material and septations is a common finding in subacute cases. USG can differentiate between thin

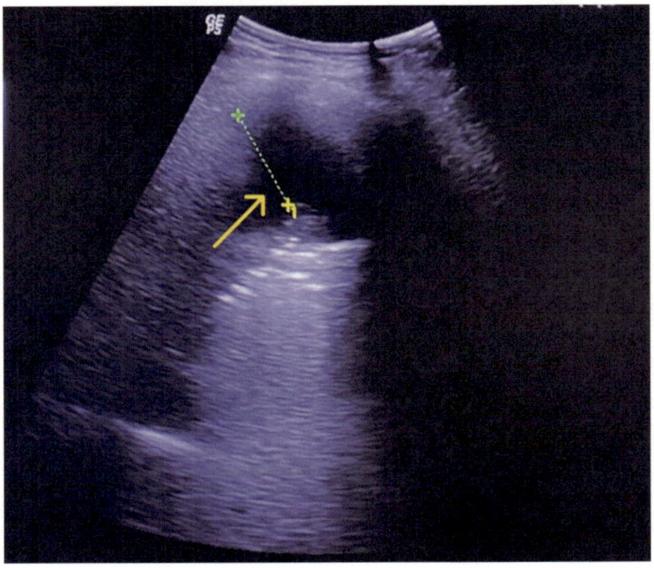

Figure 6.
USG thorax appearance of pleural effusion.

or thick septa, the presence of loculation, and thin or thick fluid based on echogenicity. It can also identify the thickening of the pleura and guide the aspiration of deep-seated effusion as well as pleural biopsy.

4.1.3 Computer tomography

A thoracic computer tomography (CT) may be necessary for further evaluation of pleural tuberculosis, especially in complicated cases. A recent study shows that the presence of subpleural nodules and septal thickening is common in patients with pulmonary tuberculosis and pleural effusion [6].

Figure 7 depicts an axial view of pleural effusion indicated by the black arrow, while **Figure 8** shows a sagittal view of pleural effusion also marked by a black arrow.

CT thorax is also helpful in detecting loculated pleural effusion and can be used for CT-guided aspiration in deep-seated pleural effusion. **Figure 9** shows a loculated pleural effusion indicated by the black arrow. Sometimes, consolidation with a cavity and pleural effusion may be detected on a CT scan of the thorax (See **Figure 10**).

4.2 Pleural fluid

Once fluid is present in the pleural space, the next step is to perform diagnostic or therapeutic thoracentesis, depending on the patient's clinical condition. The definitive diagnosis of pleural TB is made by demonstrating Mtb bacilli within the fluid. It is difficult to isolate Mtb bacilli from pleural fluid because, in the majority of cases, the fluid accumulates as a result of delayed-type hypersensitivity (DTH) to the Mtb bacilli protein. There is no test for diagnosing pleural TB with 100% sensitivity and specificity. Diagnosing TB in pleural effusion is challenging and requires consideration of clinical features, radiological findings, and laboratory investigations to confirm the diagnosis. Once fluid is aspirated, the following investigations are conducted on the pleural fluid.

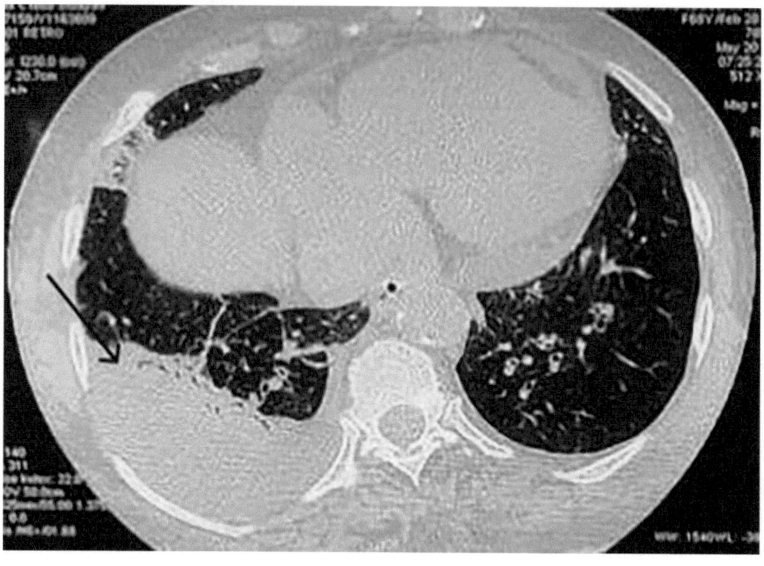

Figure 7.
Axial view of pleural effusion.

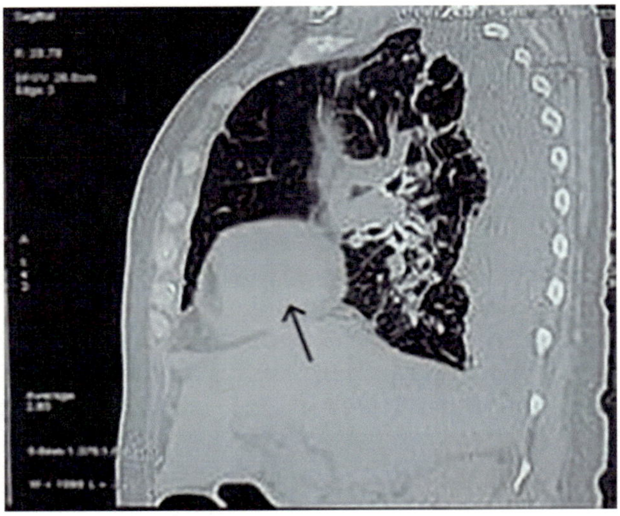

Figure 8.
Sagittal view of pleural effusion.

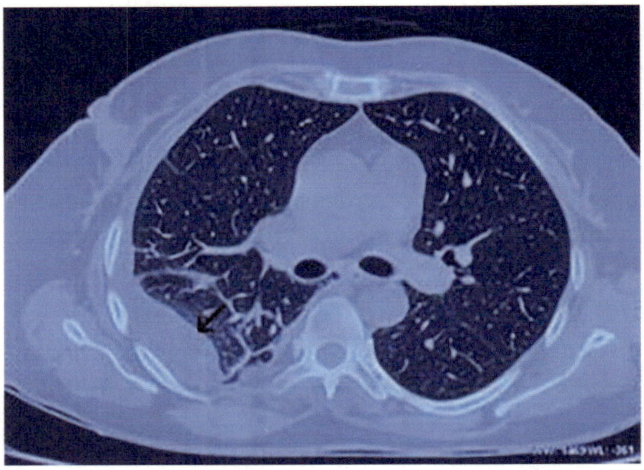

Figure 9.
Loculated pleural effusion on lateral aspect of chest wall (black arrow).

4.2.1 Total count (TC)

The total cell count (TCC) within pleural fluid is usually between 500 and 1000 cells per cubic millimeter (cmm). In pleural tuberculosis, the white blood cell count may be within the normal range or elevated. The investigation is nonspecific and may indicate other causes of pleural effusion. A high white blood cell count may raise suspicion of bacterial empyema or secondary infection in pleural TB.

4.2.2 Differential count (DC)

In pleural tuberculosis, the pleural fluid analysis within the first few days may show a neutrophilic response, followed by a predominantly lymphocytic response. Neutrophils serve as the first line of defense and respond initially. In the majority of

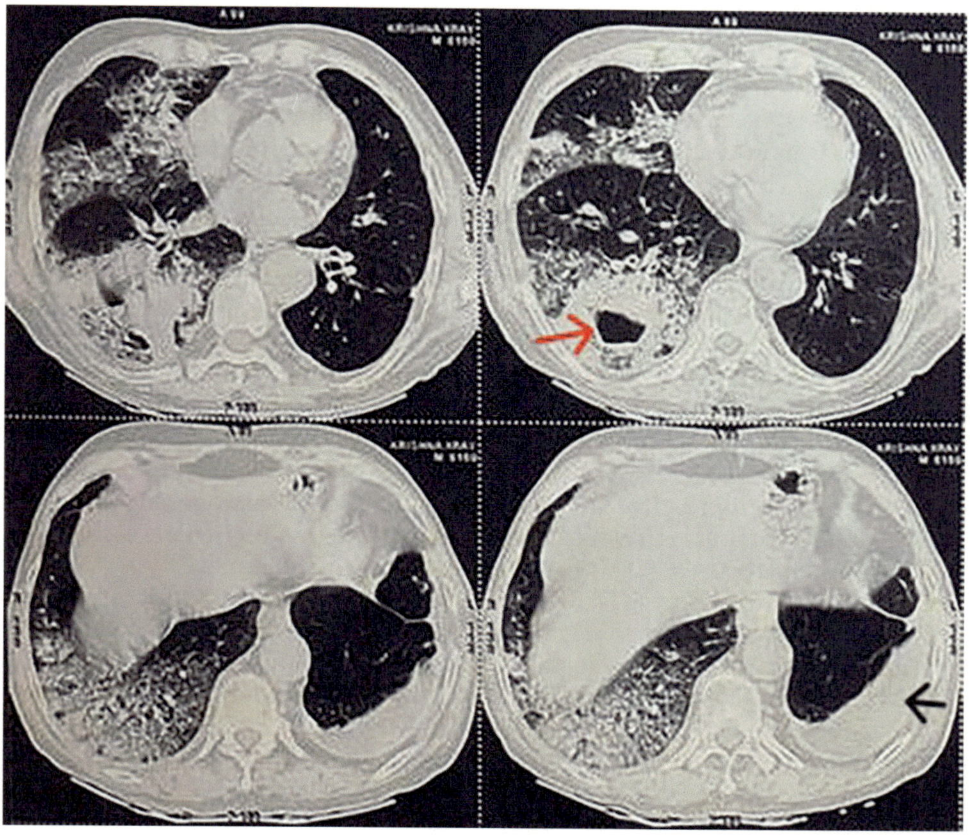

Figure 10.
Consolidation with cavity with contralateral pleural effusion.

cases, lymphocyte counts are more than 50% of the total count. Other cells that can be present include red blood cells (RBC), eosinophils, and mesothelial cells. RBCs may be present due to a traumatic tap, coexisting malignancy, or, rarely, pleural TB associated with hemorrhagic effusion. In pleural tuberculosis, there is a low number of mesothelial cells, mainly due to a decrease in shedding. Eosinophils are typically absent or present in low numbers. If there are high eosinophil levels, other possible causes need to be ruled out.

4.2.3 Biochemical analysis

The pH of the fluid is nonspecific and has no diagnostic value. The protein level in pleural tuberculosis is elevated, with levels found to be greater than 5 g/dL. The level of lactate dehydrogenase (LDH) is elevated, and once again, it is nonspecific. The levels of fluid protein and LDH, along with their serum levels, help establish the diagnosis of exudative pleural effusion using Light's criteria. The sugar level in TB pleural effusion is usually within the normal range. A low sugar level suggests a secondary bacterial infection or an alternative diagnosis other than pleural TB. Elevated sugar levels may indicate a potential diagnosis of diabetes mellitus. All the above biochemical analyses are not useful for confirming the diagnosis, but they support the diagnosis of pleural TB.

4.2.4 Adenosine deaminase (ADA) level

Elevated ADA levels are useful for diagnosing pleural TB, in addition to other fluid analyses. ADA is an enzyme involved in the catabolism of purines. Elevated levels of ADA in plasma are an indicator of stimulated cell-mediated immunity, especially T-lymphocytes. The range of ADA levels varies from 30 to 70 U/L for diagnosing pleural TB. In a study, it has been found that patients with pleural TB have ADA levels greater than 70 U/L in pleural fluid [13], while ADA levels lower than 40 U/L can rule out the diagnosis of pleural TB [13–15]. Elevated ADA levels may also be present in other conditions such as bacterial empyema, parapneumonic effusion, malignant pleural effusion, and rheumatoid pleuritis, which make it nonspecific. By using a lymphocyte-to-neutrophil ratio of 0.75 or higher in pleural fluid, the specificity of ADA can be increased [16–18]. Recently, several studies have explored the use of the LDH/ADA ratio in diagnosing pleural TB, and they have demonstrated promising results. In various studies, the sensitivity has been shown to range from 86 to 89.1% and the specificity from 84.8 to 88%, depending on the ratio value ranging from 12 to 15 [19, 20]. Other studies have also suggested that it helps differentiate between pleural TB and malignancy [21]. However, further research is needed.

There are two isomers of ADA found in the body. ADA1 is found in all cells of the body, but it is primarily present in lymphocytes, neutrophils, and monocytes [22]. The ADA1 isoenzyme is elevated in pleural effusion other than tuberculosis. The ADA2 is mainly found in monocytes and comprises 90% of the ADA raised in tuberculous pleural effusion [22]. Measurement of both isomers and the ratio of ADA1/ADA2 may help confirm the diagnosis of pleural TB.

4.2.5 Interferon gamma level

The level of Interferon Gamma in pleural fluid may be useful in diagnosing pleural TB. Interferon gamma is produced by activated macrophages and CD4+ lymphocytes in response to Mtb protein in the pleural space [23]. It is measured in pleural fluid using enzyme-linked immunosorbent assay or radioimmunoassay. A newer method, the InterGam Rapid Immuno Suspension Assay, has been developed by Antrum Biotech. This method offers increased sensitivity, specificity, and rapid turnaround time [24]. Interferon gamma levels may be elevated in empyema.

Both measuring ADA and interferon gamma levels in pleural fluid can confirm the diagnosis of pleural TB with high precision. Due to its easy availability and cost-effectiveness, ADA is the first choice for investigating pleural effusion.

4.2.6 Pleural fluid tuberculous antigen or antibody detection

In the evaluation of pleural TB, the potential use of pleural fluid TB antigen or antibody was considered, but it did not yield any promising results.

4.2.7 Other biomarker levels

Interleukin (IL) 27, lysozyme, interferon gamma-inducible 10 kDa protein, neopterin, tumor necrosis factor alpha, matrix metalloproteinase, leptin, IL-1B, IL-2, IL-12, and fibronectin levels are among the biomarkers being investigated for potential use in diagnosing pleural TB.

4.2.8 Microbiological test

As previously discussed, Mtb is difficult to isolate from pleural fluid because it results from DTH to Mtb proteins. Sometimes, direct infection of the pleura with Mtb may result in fluid accumulation, and in such cases, bacilli can be isolated.

4.2.8.1 Microscopic examination

Pleural fluid staining for acid-fast bacilli (AFB) rarely yields any results and it is positive in less than 10% of cases. A concentration of 10,000 bacilli per milliliter (mL) is required for detection under microscopy. However, pleural fluid is a paucibacillary specimen, making it difficult to diagnose based solely on microscopic examination.

4.2.8.2 Polymerase chain reaction (PCR)-based tests

4.2.8.2.1 Cartilage-based nucleic acid amplification test (CBNAAT)

CBNAAT (Xpert MTB/RIF) is a sensitive method for detecting Mtb from biological specimens. It is a PCR-based method that detects Mtb deoxyribonucleic acid from a specimen. It is a more sensitive method than microscopic evaluation because it can detect approximately 100 bacilli per milliliter. The low number of Mtb in pleural fluid makes CBNAAT less sensitive. The meta-analysis study reported a mean sensitivity of 62% and a specificity of 98% [25]. A more sensitive method, Xpert Ultra, has been developed, and it can detect up to 20 bacilli per milliliter. It is a rapid method and the turnaround time is approximately 4 hours. In addition to detecting Mtb, it also detects the presence of rifampicin drug resistance within the specimen. Recently, there is a global trend of increasing drug-resistant tuberculosis, and this test is particularly useful despite its low sensitivity. If CBNAAT does not detect Mtb, it does not rule out the diagnosis of pleural TB. In such cases, ADA or interferon gamma levels are useful in establishing the diagnosis of pleural TB.

4.2.8.2.2 Line probe assay (LPA)

LPA is a PCR-based method that can simultaneously detect resistance to rifampicin and isoniazid. Turnaround time with LPA is approximately 72 hours. Its utility in the diagnosis of pleural TB is still under investigation.

4.2.8.2.3 Culture

The culture of microorganisms is the gold standard for diagnosing infections. One drawback of PCR-based methods is their inability to differentiate between live and dead organisms. The culture method is useful not only for diagnosis but also for follow-up cases of Pleural TB.

Various culture methods are available for Mtb. The Lowenstein-Jensen medium is the most widely used and cost-effective culture method. Newer methods such as the BACTEC-Mycobacteria Growth Indicator Tube (MGIT) are more rapid than the solid culture method and have a higher yield [26, 27].

In individuals with HIV, there is a high possibility of pleural fluid testing positive for acid-fast bacilli (AFB) and the isolation of Mtb on culture [28, 29]. If the CD4 count is less than 100 cells per mL^{-1}, there is an increased possibility of AFB-positive pleural fluid [28].

4.3 Pleural biopsy

If pleural fluid analysis is non-diagnostic or if there is a need to rule out other causes, pleural biopsy is helpful in such situations. PCR-based methods can be used in pleural biopsy specimens and have identical or superior sensitivity compared to histopathological examination. It is prudent to use a combination of microbiological, histopathological, and PCR-based methods for the evaluation of pleural TB [30].

4.3.1 Transcutaneous closed pleural biopsy

A closed biopsy is taken from the pleura, either after marking the site using ultrasound of the thorax or under the guidance of thoracic ultrasound. There are various methods to use for biopsy.

4.3.1.1 Abram's or cope needle

Both biopsy needles can be used blindly or under USG thorax guidance. The specimen is mainly obtained from the parietal pleura and multiple passes at multiple sites yield better results. The procedure is performed under local anesthesia and requires skill to conduct a biopsy. The bore of the needle is wider and may result in complications such as local pain, secondary infection, hemothorax, and pneumothorax. The rate of complications may be lower when using USG or CT guidance.

4.3.1.2 Automatic Bart biopsy gun

This gun is easy to operate due to its simplicity. It can be used blindly or under guidance. Its complication rate is the same as that of the above-mentioned needle.

4.3.2 Thoracoscopy/pleuroscopy

Pleural biopsy is obtained via thoracoscopy or pleuroscopy under direct visualization. Tubercles can be identified scattered over the parietal/visceral pleura, as well as septa within the pleural space, and biopsies can be taken. Sometimes, a parietal pleural biopsy may show no signs of pleural TB. In such cases, a visceral pleural biopsy may yield a diagnosis [31].

The pleural biopsy specimen can be used for microbiological examination, histopathological analysis, and culture. Staining of a pleural biopsy for AFB may show the organism in less than 10% of cases when no granuloma is present in the biopsy [4, 32]. Histopathological examination reveals granulomas within the biopsy of pleural TB, but granulomas may also be present in other conditions such as rheumatoid pleuritis, sarcoidosis, fungal infections, and sometimes in malignancy. Tuberculous granuloma is characterized by necrotizing caseating granulomas as caseous necrosis is not characteristic of other granulomatous inflammation. When pleural biopsy is used in conjunction with culture and histopathological examination, it can increase the chances of diagnosing pleural TB up to 95% [33].

4.4 Other

4.4.1 Sputum examination

Cough in cases of pleural effusion is usually dry, so it has no diagnostic value. When pleural effusion is associated with parenchymal lesions and a productive cough, sputum examination may detect Mtb using staining or molecular techniques, as mentioned above.

4.4.2 Tuberculin skin test

It is also known as the Mantoux test (MT). It has no diagnostic value in endemic areas where the prevalence of latent TB is high. When all investigations are inconclusive, the result of MT may support the diagnosis of TB. This test only indicates infection with Mtb but not the presence of the disease.

4.4.3 Interferon gamma release assay (IGRA)

The IGRA test measures the level of interferon gamma in response to stimulation with tuberculous antigen in the patient's serum. As with MT, it has no diagnostic value in endemic areas and cannot identify disease, only infection. Both tests are useful in areas where the prevalence of TB is low.

Due to the paucibacillary nature of pleural effusion and the lack of a sensitive test for pleural TB, a definitive diagnosis is not made in many cases.

5. Treatment

Once a diagnosis of pleural TB is made based on clinical, microscopic, or molecular methods, the next step is to start anti-tuberculous drugs.

5.1 Anti-tuberculous treatment

Anti-tuberculous drugs are the mainstay of treatment for pleural TB. If PCR-based methods are used for evaluation and yield inconclusive results or confirm drug-sensitive Mtb, a combination of isoniazid, rifampicin, ethambutol, and pyrazinamide is suggested. The combination of these four drugs is administered for 2 months, followed by 4 months of isoniazid, rifampicin, and ethambutol [34]. Pleural TB in HIV patients remains the same as in non-HIV patients. The response to the treatment is indicated by the resolution of fever, a decrease in the frequency and severity of cough, a reduction in the severity of chest pain, and an improvement in appetite. These changes are usually noticed within 2 weeks of treatment. The resolution of pleural fluid occurs within 6 to 12 weeks after starting treatment, depending on the amount of fluid, presence of septation, and associated comorbidities such as DM.

If a PCR-based method suggests drug-resistant tuberculosis, the choice of drugs is based on the pattern of drug resistance identified by the PCR-based method and the results of the drug sensitivity test (DST) culture. The combination of drugs and duration of treatment varies according to the geographic area and the prevalence of drug-resistant tuberculosis.

5.2 Anti-inflammatory drugs

Corticosteroid treatment is not recommended for pleural TB. In certain situations, when patients experience severe symptoms such as chest pain, fever, or breathlessness that interfere with their daily lives, corticosteroids are administered. If necessary, it should be administered along with anti-tuberculous drugs at a dose of 0.5–0.75 milligrams per kilogram, followed by rapid tapering [8].

Serratiopeptidase is a proteolytic enzyme that possesses anti-inflammatory, anti-fibrotic, and analgesic properties [35]. The role of the anti-inflammatory drug serratiopeptidase has been shown to improve clinical outcomes and avoid surgery in cases of hydropneumothorax caused by tuberculosis, when used in conjunction with anti-tubercular drugs [35]. However, its study in pleural effusion is lacking. In certain situations, when corticosteroid use is contraindicated, and there are high TC in pleural fluid and severe symptoms, this drug may be useful. However, further studies are required.

5.3 Surgery

Surgery plays a limited role in the management of pleural TB. Surgical management in the form of thoracentesis or insertion of an intercostal drainage tube (ICD) may be necessary. Thoracentesis may be required in patients with a large effusion and shortness of breath to relieve symptoms. When thoracentesis is used in conjunction with anti-tuberculous drugs and corticosteroids, faster resolution of symptoms occurs [36, 37].

ICD insertion is necessary in cases of massive pleural effusion requiring immediate relief, pus formation, or failure to resolve due to excessive septation within the pleural cavity. The use of intrapleural fibrinolytic drugs is beneficial in terms of rapid drainage and resolution on chest radiograph, improvement in symptoms, reduction in the time from treatment to drainage, and improvement in forced vital capacity and total lung capacity at the end of treatment [38–42]. Fibrinolytic drugs primarily break down septa and liquefy fluid, resulting in the rapid clearance of fluid.

Thoracoscopy is required when pleural TB is complicated by loculated pleural effusion, thickened calcified pleura, pus formation, and excessive septa that do not respond to fibrinolytic therapy.

5.4 Follow-up

Follow-up of patients with pleural TB is required to evaluate the resolution of symptoms, the resolution of pleural fluid, and any adverse effects of anti-tuberculous treatment. If resolution of symptoms or pleural fluid does not occur, then alternative or additional diagnoses need to be investigated.

6. Complications

Residual pleural thickening is the most common complication found in patients with pleural TB. More than 2 mm of residual remains visible on the chest radiograph and CT scan after 24 weeks of treatment [35]. Fibrothorax is a severe form of thickening that occurs when pleural TB remains inadequately treated, untreated, or in patients with TB empyema. Calcification of residual pleural thickening may be noticed on chest radiographs. Due to residual pleural thickening, the patient may experience intermittent or persistent chest pain on the side of the effusion. Restrictive pulmonary function abnormalities may occur in such patients. Decortication is necessary in severe cases to alleviate restrictive changes. TB empyema may develop as a complication of pleural TB or as a distinct entity.

7. Conclusion

Pleural TB is the second most common extra-pulmonary form of tuberculosis, following TB lymphadenitis. Pleural TB is most likely to occur due to the rupture of a subpleural caseous focus within the lung or sometimes due to the spread of infection from a lymph node into the pleural space. DTH is a mechanism by which fluid accumulates within the pleural space, but it is rarely due to direct infection with Mtb. It is a disease that affects the young population. The presentation may be acute to subacute and symptoms can range from pleuritic chest pain, nonproductive cough, anorexia, weight loss, night sweats, and dyspnea in severe cases. Evaluation methods include radiological imaging, pleural fluid analysis using molecular and culture methods, pleural biopsy, and sputum examination. Anti-tuberculosis drugs are the mainstay of treatment and the choice depends upon DST results. Thoracentesis and ICD insertion may be required in severe cases. Residual pleural biopsy is the most common form of complication.

Conflict of interest

The authors declare no conflict of interest.

Other declarations

Images are original, prepared by author and previously unpublished.

Author details

Yagnang Vyas
Dr. N.D. Desai Faculty of Medical Science and Research, Dharmsinh Desai University, Nadiad, Gujarat, India

*Address all correspondence to: yagnang@gmail.com

References

[1] Baumann MH, Nolan R, Petrini M, Lee YC, Light RW, Schneider E. Pleural tuberculosis in the United States: Incidence and drug resistance. Chest. 2007;**131**:1125-1132

[2] Diacon AH, Van de Wal BW, Wyser C, Smedema JP, Bezuidenhout J, Bolliger CT, et al. Diagnostic tools in tuberculous pleurisy: A direct comparative study. The European Respiratory Journal. 2003;**22**:589-591

[3] Udwadia ZF, Sen T. Pleural tuberculosis: An update. Current Opinion in Pulmonary Medicine. 2010;**16**(4):399-406. DOI: 10.1097/MCP.0b013e328339cf6e

[4] Berger HW, Mejia E. Tuberculous pleurisy. Chest. 1973;**63**:88-92

[5] Stead WW, Eichenholz A, Stauss HK. Operative and pathologic findings in twenty-four patients with syndrome of idiopathic pleurisy with effusion, presumably tuberculous. American Review of Tuberculosis. 1955;**71**:473-502

[6] Jung MK et al. CT scan differences of pulmonary TB according to presence of pleural effusion. Chest. 2023;**164**(6):1387-1395

[7] Light RW. Tuberculous pleural effusions. In: Light RW, editor. Pleural Diseases. Philadelphia: Williams & Wilkins; 1995

[8] Light RW. Update on tuberculous pleural effusion. Respirology. 2010;**15**:451-458

[9] Jones BE, Young SMM, Antoniskis D, Davidson PT, Kramer F, Barnes PF. Relationship of the manifestations of tuberculosis to CD4 cell counts in patients with human immunodeficiency virus infection. The American Review of Respiratory Disease. 1993;**148**:1292-1297

[10] Frye MD, Pozsik CJ, Sahn SA. Tuberculous pleurisy is more common in AIDS than in non-AIDS patients with tuberculosis. Chest. 1997;**112**:393-397

[11] Andreu J, Caceres J, Pallisa E, et al. Radiological manifestations of pulmonary tuberculosis. European Journal of Radiology. 2004;**51**(2):139-149

[12] Valdes L, Alvarez D, San Jose E, et al. Tuberculous pleurisy: A study of 254 patients. Archives of Internal Medicine. 1998;**158**(18):2017-2021

[13] Ocana I, Martinez-Vazquez JM, Segura RM, et al. Adenosine deaminase in pleural fluids: Test for diagnosis of tuberculous pleural effusion. Chest. 1983;**84**:51-53

[14] Fontan Bueso J, Verea Hernando H, Garcia-Buela JP, Dominguez Juncal L, Martin Egana MT, Montero Martinez MC. Diagnostic value of simultaneous determination of pleural adenosine deaminase and pleural lysozyme/serum lysozyme ratio in pleural effusions. Chest. 1988;**93**:303-307

[15] Valdes L, San Jose E, Alvarez D, Sarandeses A, Pose A, Chomon B, et al. Diagnosis of tuberculous pleurisy using the biologic parameters adenosine deaminase, lysozyme, and interferon gamma. Chest. 1993;**103**:458-465

[16] Burgess LJ, Maritz FJ, Le Roux I, et al. Combined use of pleural adenosine deaminase with lymphocyre/neutrophil ratio. Increased specificity for the diagnosis of tuberculous pleuritis. Chest. 1996;**109**:414-419

[17] Valdes L, San Jose MA, Pose A, e t al. Diagnosing tuberculous pleural effusion using clinical data and pleural fluid analysis. A study of patients less than 40 years-old in an area with a high incidence of tuberculosis. Respiratory Medicine. 2010;**104**:1211-1217

[18] Diacon AH, Van de Wal BW, Wyser C, et al. Diagnostic tools in tuberculous pleurisy: A direct comparative study. The European Respiratory Journal. 2003;**22**:589-591

[19] Blakiston M, Chiu W, Wong C, et al. Diagnostic performance of pleural fluid adenosine deaminase for tuberculous pleural effusion in a low-incidence setting. Journal of Clinical Microbiology. 2018;**56**(8):e00258-e00218. DOI: 10.1128/JCM.00258-18

[20] Beukes A, Shaw JA, Diacon AH, et al. The utility of pleural fluid lactate dehydrogenase to adenosine deaminase ratio in pleural tuberculosis. Respiration. 2020;**100**:59-63. DOI: 10.1159/000509555

[21] Wang J, Liu J, Xie X, et al. The pleural fluid lactate dehydrogenase/adenosine deaminase ratio differentiates between tuberculous and parapneumonic pleural effusions. BMC Pulmonary Medicine. 2017;**17**(1):168

[22] Perez-Rodriguez E, Castro DJ. The use of ADA and ADA isoenzymes in the diagnosis of tuberculous pleuritis. Current Opinion in Pulmonary Medicine. 2000;**6**:259-266

[23] Barnes PF, Mistry SD, Cooper CL, et al. Compartmentalization of a CD4+ T lymphocyte subpopulation in tuberculous pleuritis. Journal of Immunology. 1989;**142**:1114-1119

[24] Meldau R, Randall P, Pooran A, et al. Same-day tools, including Xpert ultra and IRISA-TB, for rapid diagnosis of pleural tuberculosis: A prospective observational study. Journal of Clinical Microbiology. 2019;**57**(9):e00614-e00619

[25] Pai M, Flores LL, Hubbard A, et al. Nucleic acid amplification tests in the diagnosis of tuberculous pleuritis: A systematic review and meta-analysis. BMC Infectious Diseases. 2004;**4**:1-14

[26] Ruan S-Y, Chuang Y-C, Wang J-Y, et al. Revisiting tuberculous pleurisy: Pleural fluid characteristics and diagnostic yield of mycobacterial culture in an endemic area. Thorax. 2012;**67**(9):822-827

[27] von Groote-Bidlingmaier F, Koegelenberg CF, Bolliger CT, et al. The yield of different pleural fluid volumes for *Mycobacterium tuberculosis* culture. Thorax. 2013;**68**(3):290-291. DOI: 10.1136/thoraxjnl-2012-202338

[28] Heyderman RS, Makunike R, Muza T, et al. Pleural tuberculosis in Harare, Zimbabwe: The relationship between human immunodeficiency virus, CD4 lymphocyte count, granuloma formation and disseminated disease. Tropical Medicine & International Health. 1998;**3**:14-20

[29] Luzze H, Elliott AM, Joloba ML, et al. Evaluation of suspected tuberculous pleurisy: Clinical and diagnostic findings in HIV- I -positive and HIV-negative adults in Uganda. The International Journal of Tuberculosis and Lung Disease. 2001;**5**:746-753

[30] Hasaneen NA, Zaki ME, Shalaby HM, El-Morsi AS. Polymerase chain reaction of pleural biopsy is a rapid and sensitive method for the diagnosis of tuberculous pleural effusion. Chest. 2003;**124**:2105-2111

[31] Jain NK, Guhan AR, Joshi N, Dixit R, Singh V, Meena RP. Comparative study

of visceral and parietal pleural biopsy in the etiological diagnosis of pleural diseases. The Journal of the Association of Physicians of India. 2000;**48**:776-780

[32] Kim JS, Shim SS, Kim Y, Ryu YJ, Lee JH. Chest CT findings of pleural tuberculosis: Differential diagnosis of pleural tuberculosis and malignant pleural dissemination. Acta Radiologica. 2014;**55**:1063-1068

[33] Prakash UB, Reiman HM. Comparison of needle biopsy with cytologic analysis for the evaluation of pleural effusion: Analysis of 414 cases. Mayo Clinic Proceedings. 1985;**60**:158-164

[34] Technical and Operational Guidelines for TB Control in India 2016: Central TB Division [Internet]. Available from: https://tbcindia.gov.in/index1.php?lang=1&level=2&sublinkid=4573&lid=3177 [Accessed: June 16, 2023]

[35] Shukla AD, Agarwal V. Does serratiopeptidase prevent thoracic surgery in patients of hydropneumothorax of tubercular aetiology. Lung India. 2023;**40**(5):445-448. DOI: 10.4103/lungindia.lungindia_109_23

[36] Galarza I, Canete C, Granados A, et al. Randomised trial of corticosteroids in the treatment of tuberculous pleurisy. Thorax. 1995;**50**:1305-1307

[37] Wyser C, Walz G, Smedema JP, et al. Corticosteroids in the treatment of tuberculous pleurisy. A double-blind, placebocontrolled, randomized study. Chest. 1996;**110**:333-338

[38] Cao G-Q, Li L, Wang Y-B, et al. Treatment of free flowing tuberculous pleurisy with intrapleural urokinase. The International Journal of Tuberculosis and Lung Disease. 2015;**19**(11):1395-1400

[39] Barthwal MS, Marwah V, Chopra M, et al. A Fiveyear study of intrapleural fibrinolytic therapy in loculated pleural collections. The Indian Journal of Chest Diseases & Allied Sciences. 2016;**58**(1):17-20

[40] Meghji J, Simpson H, Squire SB, et al. A systematic review of the prevalence and pattern of imaging defined post-TB lung disease. PLoS One. 2016;**11**(8):e0161176

[41] Jantz MA, Antony VB. Pleural fibrosis. Clinics in Chest Medicine. 2006;**27**(2):181-191

[42] Candela A, Andujar J, Hernandez L, et al. Functional sequelae of tuberculous pleurisy in patients correctly treated. Chest. 2003;**123**(6):1996-2000

Section 3

Mesothelioma

Chapter 4

Malignant Pleural Mesothelioma

Nishant Allena, Sindhaghatta Venkatram
and Gilda Diaz-Fuentes

Abstract

Malignant pleural mesothelioma is a rare tumor with a dismal prognosis that originates in the mesothelial surfaces of the pleura. The main risk factor is exposure to asbestos. Worldwide, especially in developed countries, occupational asbestos exposure has decreased significantly. Due to the long latency between exposure and development of mesothelioma, the disease is still very relevant and cases are seen sporadically. Despite advances in diagnostic imaging and clinical research, early and prompt diagnosis is challenging. Some serum tumor markers are promising but not incorporated to guidelines yet. Current treatments have been evolving very slowly in recent years; treatment focus in the use of chemotherapy, radiation and surgery. This chapter aims to present a review of malignant pleural mesothelioma to assist the practicing physician in the early recognition and evaluation of patients presenting with suspected pleural mesothelioma.

Keywords: malignant mesothelioma, asbestos, pleural disease, pleural tumor, environmental tumor

1. Introduction

Malignant mesothelioma (MM) is a rare, highly aggressive and fatal disease which originates in the mesothelial surfaces of pleura or, rarely, in other serosal membranes such as peritoneum, pericardium, and tunica vaginalis [1]. Most cases of MM have been linked to asbestos exposure. Some studies confirmed asbestos exposure in up to 80% to −86% of patients with MM; latency period between first between the first exposure and tumor development, is long and ranges from 15 to 60 years [2, 3].

Malignant pleural mesothelioma (MPM) is the most common type seen in up to 70% of cases, followed by peritoneal and pericardial mesothelioma in 30% and 1–2% respectively.

The survival of patients with mesothelioma is the worst compared with all the other types of cancer; this is related to the stage at diagnosis which is usually advanced and lack of new more effective therapies for treatment. Reported survival for mesothelioma is a 5-year survival rate of less than 10% and a median survival time of less than 1 year. In patients with early stage of MPM, overall survival is better compared with those diagnosed at a late stage; 5-year survival ranges between 7% and 24% [4–8].

2. Epidemiology and pathogenesis

The incidence of malignant pleural mesothelioma (MPM) is low and it has been reported to be less than 5/100,000 inhabitants in Europe [9]. The World Health Organization estimates that as many as 92,250 people die annually per year worldwide due to asbestos-related disease with around 43,000 dying of mesothelioma; more than 80% are related to occupational exposure [4, 5]. The continued use of asbestos products in developing countries raises concern of an increased incidence of MPM in the future and there are predictions that incidence will continue increasing until 2030 [10].

Other factors linking to predisposition for MM includes a germline mutation in the BAP1 gene, somatic mutations, ionizing radiation such as in patients previously treated with radiotherapy, exposure to erionite (which may be found in travel roads). Smoking has not been reported to be a risk factor for MM [11].

Several report suggest an increased risk for MPM in people exposed to asbestos who develop benign asbestos pleural diseases like pleural plaques; other investigators did not find same relationship in people with asbestos related pleural thickening [12–14].

Detailed review of the potential molecular mechanisms underlying the pathogenesis of asbestos-related diseases and mesothelioma is out of the scope of this review. Several studies suggest that asbestos fibers deposited in lungs and translocated to the pleura could have direct genotoxic effects on epithelial and mesothelial cells.

Generation of reactive oxygen and nitric species leading to oxidative stress and chronic inflammation is the main molecular mechanism linking asbestos exposure with the development of fibroplasia and neoplasia. Reactive oxygen species can be generated directly by the asbestos fibers or indirectly by inflammatory cell which will lead to release of cytokines that will potentiate the inflammatory response [15, 16]. Asbestos fibers have been shown to induce chromosomal and genetic damage in mammalian cells; mesothelioma is characterized by multiple chromosomal alterations [17, 18].

Studies suggest that the main mechanisms in the development of fibrosis and malignant cell transformation in patients exposed to asbestos are chronic inflammation, oxidative stress, genetic and epigenetic changes and direct cellular toxicity and genotoxicity [19].

3. Diagnosis and clinical presentation

Diagnosis of MPM is challenging as usually symptoms are non-specific, they can develop slowly over a period of months and many times information regarding asbestos exposure is not readily available. Patients tend to present with advanced disease and at advanced age, the average age for a MPM presentation is 72.

Symptoms are usually related to the extension of the disease and ranges from dyspnea, thoracic pain and constitutional symptoms to life threatening conditions like superior vena cava syndrome or pericardial tamponade due to malignancy [20, 21]. See **Table 1** for details of symptoms [25].

Due to the vague symptoms diagnosis delays are not unusual as symptoms can be attributed to other pathologies. A very detailed occupational and medical history is necessary to identify exposure to asbestos and other potential predisposing risk factors.

Symptoms	Comments
Constitutional symptoms	Weight loss, fatigue, anorexia, low grade-fever
Dyspnea-usually chronic	Due to pleural effusion
Cough-dry	Reported in up to 10% of patients [22, 23]
Thoracic pain	Unilateral, constant, dull, irradiation to shoulder or upper abdomen due to pleural irritation
Dysphagia	Due to esophageal compression
Neurological symptoms	Sympathetic nerve involvement of the arm with neuropathic pain and Pancoast tumor symptoms, Horners's syndrome, recurrent laryngeal nerve palsy due to tumor invasion
Intermittent hypoglycemia	Multifactorial—secretion of insulinase inhibitor [24], secretion of leucine like substance stimulating insulin release

Table 1.
Clinical presentation of malignant pleural mesothelioma.

Unexplained pleural pain associated with pleural effusion in subjects with asbestos exposure should raise concern for MPM; more than 70% of patients with MPM develop malignant pleural effusion [26].

An accurate and expedited diagnosis is important. Diagnostic investigation include initial non-invasive investigation with chest radiographs, high resolution computed tomogram of the chest (HRCT), occasionally Magnetic Resonance Imaging (MRI), Positron emission tomography computed tomogram (PET-CT) among others [27]. Cytological and tissue diagnosis is needed for diagnosis and management. Several serum tumor markers have been investigated to help in early diagnosis but their diagnostic role is still under investigation [3, 28–30]. Another promising diagnostics technique are the analysis of exhaled breath of patients with mesothelioma to evaluate volatile organic compounds and circulating tumor cells test (liquid biopsy [31, 32]. See **Table 2** for details.

Definitive diagnosis of MPM requires histopathology, supported by clinic-radiological findings.

3.1 Imaging modalities

3.1.1 X-ray

Chest X-rays are the primary imaging method used to detect suspicious features indicative of malignant pleural mesothelioma.

Pleural effusion is observed in 70% of cases [26], along with pleural plaques, pleural thickening, and interstitial lung disease, which are suggestive of asbestosis. Additionally, blunting of the costophrenic angle due to small effusions or pleural thickening, as well as a reduction in hemithorax size, may also be present.

3.1.2 Computed tomography

Computed tomography (CT) plays a pivotal role in the diagnosis and management of MPM. CT imaging provides detailed anatomical information and is crucial for assessing the extent of disease involvement, guiding treatment decisions, and

Modality	Common findings	Advantages	Disadvantages
Non-invasive evaluation			
Chest radiograph	Pleural effusion Nodular pleural thickening or masses Pneumothorax (rare) Pericardial effusion	Inexpensive Readily available	Poor sensitivity to detect small pleural effusion or pleural disease
HRCT (high resolution computed tomography) chest	Pleural effusion/thickening/masses Interlobular, lobular, mediastinal and parietal pleural thickening Involvement of interlobar fissure Chest wall involvement Pneumothorax (rare) Pericardial effusion	Sensitive to detect pulmonary and pericardial disease	
MRI (Magnetic Resonance Imaging)	As HRCT of chest with better resolutions to evaluate neurological and soft tissue involvement	Good to evaluate tumor expansion and superior soft tissue contrast Good to evaluate neurological complications of tumor	Expensive, not readily available, radiology reading expertise needed
PET-CT (Positron Imaging Tomography Scan) chest	Unilateral circumferential pleural and fissural thickening with ^{18}F-FDG avidity	Useful for staging and treatment response	Cannot differentiate between MPM versus other malignant pleural effusion
Serum tumor markers	Mesothelin Fibulin-3 Osteopontin HMGB-1 (high mobility group box 1)	Potential to support diagnosis	Studies are not consistent Under investigation
• Volatile organic compounds in exhaled breath • Liquid biopsy		Non invasive	Still investigational
Invasive evaluation			
Pleural fluid analysis/cytology	Usually negative or inconclusive	Immediate therapeutic relief in cases of large volume effusions	Low sensitivity
Pleural biopsy	Histopathology showing cells characteristic of the type of mesothelioma	High sensitivity and specificity	Longer hospital length of stay post procedure and post op pain

Table 2.
Diagnosis of malignant pleural mesothelioma.

monitoring response to therapy. By delineating the characteristic features of MPM, such as pleural thickening, effusion, and other associated findings, CT scans are essential for accurate diagnosis and staging of this challenging disease. Main radiological findings in patients with MPM are described in **Table 2**, parietal pleural thickening exceeding 1 cm, and circumferential pleural thickening are highly suggestive of

MPM. In one study of 219 cases, pleural thickening was observed in 90%, diffuse in 63%, nodular in 22%, and mass-type in 7%. Interesting, pleural effusion was present in 79% of cases, and mediastinal lymphadenopathy in 25% [33].

3.1.3 Magnetic Resonance Imaging

Magnetic Resonance Imaging (MRI) has emerged as a valuable imaging tool in the assessment of MPM, offering unique advantages over other modalities such as CT and PET. By providing detailed soft tissue contrast and multiplanar imaging capabilities, MRI can enhance the detection, characterization, and staging of MPM, aiding in treatment planning and prognostication. When MRI was compared with chest CT in patients with MPM, MRI was better in patients with small foci, and to differentiate malignant from benign disease [34, 35]. MRI is an important study to evaluate loco-regional involvement of MPM due to the high soft tissues contrast and resolution [36]. MRI is important to investigate the resectability of pleural tumors and to plan surgery in selected patients. Studies have shown that peak tumor enhancement on MRI occurs between 150 and 300 seconds following intravenous (IV) contrast administration and hence delayed phase MRI imaging is recommended [37].

3.1.4 Positron Imaging Tomography Scan

PET scanning has emerged as a valuable tool in the diagnosis and management of MPM. By detecting metabolic activity in tissues, PET scans provide functional information that complements the anatomical details obtained from other imaging modalities like CT scans and MRI. This non-invasive imaging technique allows for more accurate staging, assessment of treatment response, and monitoring of disease progression in MPM patients. FDG PET has diagnostic and prognostic importance, it can identify metabolically active areas which can be correlated with imaging information, it may locate best areas for tissue biopsies and may predict prognosis in patients during treatment. A higher FDG uptake has been associated with shorter survival [38, 39].

3.2 Biomarkers

In recent years, there has been growing interest in the use of biomarkers as valuable tools for improving the early detection, prognostication, and monitoring of MPM. Biomarkers are measurable indicators of biological processes or responses to treatment, and their identification and validation hold promise for enhancing the clinical management of MPM. Currently, three blood biomarkers have potential for the diagnosis of MPM and include soluble mesothelin related proteins (SMRP), Osteopontin and Fibulin-3.

3.2.1 Soluble mesothelin related peptides

Soluble mesothelin-related peptides (SMRPs) are normally present in mesothelin cells but show increased expression in various cancer types. These peptides are associated with the cell membrane and undergo processing to produce both megakaryocyte-potentiating factor (MPF) and mesothelin. Mesothelin contributes to the survival and growth of tumor cells by activating the NF-kB pathway [40]. Studies by Hollevoet and colleagues conducted on a population of 4491 participants of which 1026 had a diagnosis of MPM and 3465 were controls (healthy, healthy asbestos exposed, benign asbestos related disease, benign respiratory disease and lung cancer) [41] have demonstrated that mesothelin, when used as a diagnostic marker, exhibits a high specificity of 96% but a relatively lower sensitivity of 47%. Importantly, levels of SMRPs have been found to inversely correlate with overall survival, as reported in their research. While it could be elevated in ovarian, pancreatic adenocarcinoma and parenchymal lung tumors a study by Creany et al. [42] reinforced its sensitivity by showing that SMRP was positive in only 2.8% and 1.6% in other malignancies and non malignant lung and pleural diseases respectively.

3.2.2 Osteopontin

Osteopontin is an extracellular cell adhesion protein known for its role in mediating cell-matrix interactions and cell signaling through interaction with integrin and CD44 receptors. It has been found to be elevated in a wide range of malignancies including neurological, gastrointestinal, lung, breast and bladder cancer. In a seminal study by Pass et al. [43], it was found that serum levels of osteopontin were significantly elevated in patients diagnosed with pleural mesothelioma compared to individuals with a history of asbestos exposure ($P < 0.001$). Specifically, using a cutoff value of 48.3 ng/mL, the receiver operating characteristic (ROC) curve analysis revealed a sensitivity of 77.6% and a specificity of 85.5% when comparing the group exposed to asbestos with the group diagnosed with mesothelioma.

3.2.3 Fibulin-3

Fibulin-3, a conserved member of the fibulin family of extracellular glycoproteins encoded by the EFEMP1 gene, has been the focus of recent research. In a study conducted by Pass et al. comparing patients with malignant pleural mesothelioma (MPM) and those with only asbestos exposure, higher levels of plasma fibulin-3 were observed in the MPM group. The causes of non-mesothelioma effusions ranged from congestive heart failure, adenocarcinoma and squamous cell carcinomas of the lung and also lymphoma. High levels of fibulin-3 have been found in pleural effusions of patients with MPM when compared to those patients with pleural effusion unrelated to MPM. A cutoff value of 52.8 ng/mL for levels of plasma fibulin-3 showed a sensitivity of 96.7% and a specificity of 95.5% in distinguishing patients with MPM from those without [29].

3.2.4 HMGB1

HMGB1, a well-known damage-associated molecular pattern (DAMP), plays a crucial role in inflammation. Studies have revealed that the total level of HMGB1 in the blood was notably elevated in both MPM patients and individuals exposed to asbestos, in comparison to healthy controls [44]. It is also found in lymphomas and lung cancers. Patients with MPM had higher levels of HMGB1 when compared to asbestos-exposed individuals and healthy controls. A cutoff value of 2.0 ng/mL for serum hyperacetylated HMGB1 showed a sensitivity and specificity of 100% in distinguishing patients with MPM from controls or exposed to asbestos [44].

3.3 Invasive modalities

3.3.1 Thoracentesis

Thoracentesis serves as the primary invasive diagnostic and therapeutic intervention, albeit offering only symptomatic relief, for patients presenting with a large pleural effusion as the primary symptom of MPM. Its sensitivity ranges between 16% and 30.8% [45] due to the challenge of differentiating between reactive mesothelial cells and malignant cells. Furthermore, in addition to its pivotal role in diagnosing malignant pleural effusion (MPE), thoracentesis plays a central role in palliative treatment by facilitating the drainage of a substantial volume of pleural fluid.

3.3.2 Video Assisted Thoracoscopic Surgery

With its minimally invasive nature, Video Assisted Thoracoscopic Surgery (VATS) offers several advantages over traditional open surgery, including reduced postoperative pain, shorter hospital stays, and quicker recovery times. In the context of MPM, VATS plays a crucial role in both diagnosis and treatment, allowing for precise tissue sampling and the performance of various therapeutic procedures.

Performing pleural biopsy via VATS provides the advantage of visualizing and precisely sampling representative areas from different sites within the pleural cavity. This approach allows for the retrieval of larger tissue samples, significantly enhancing the probability of confirming the diagnosis [46]. Additionally, VATS enables thorough drainage of any pleural effusion and comprehensive exploration of the entire thoracic cavity, facilitating the assessment of disease extent. Additionally, positive-pressure ventilation under direct observation after the procedure enables the evaluation of lung re-expansion following effusion drainage, informing subsequent management strategies [47]. VATS pleural biopsy is generally well-tolerated, with patients typically experiencing minimal post operative pain and a short hospital stay.

VATS pleural biopsies demonstrate a sensitivity of 95%, specificity of 100%, and negative predictive value of 94% [48]. These diagnostic performance metrics are comparable to those of medical thoracoscopy, although no randomized trial has directly compared the two procedures. Notably, VATS also offers the advantage of facilitating more invasive surgical interventions, such as lung resection and tumor debulking, concurrently with the diagnostic procedure.

3.4 Histopathology

MPM shows diverse histological subtypes: epithelioid (60–80%), sarcomatoid (<10%), and biphasic/mixed (10–15%) [49]. Epithelioid MPM displays various histological patterns with polygonal, oval, or cuboidal cells resembling reactive mesothelial cells. Mitotic activity is generally low but can be higher in poorly differentiated cases [46]. Sarcomatoid MPM is rare but aggressive, characterized by spindle-shaped cells with varying nuclear atypia and mitotic activity [50]. Heterologous differentiation, such as osteoid or bone formation, is uncommon. Biphasic MPM contains both epithelioid and sarcomatoid components, each comprising at least 10% of the tumor. If one component is less than 10%, the tumor may be predominantly classified as either sarcomatoid or epithelioid [51]. While metastatic lesions also present with atypical features, the histopathology depends on primary site of origin and diagnosis is mainly dependent on Immunohistochemical (IHC) staining.

3.4.1 Role of BRCA associated protein 1 (BAP-1) immunohistochemistry

Differentiating between malignant mesothelioma and reactive mesothelial proliferation can pose significant challenges in both histology and cytology. The loss of the BAP1 protein is a common occurrence in mesothelioma, particularly in the epithelioid/biphasic subtypes, often linked to homozygous BAP1 deletion. BAP1 immunostaining from pleural fluid serves as an outstanding biomarker, exhibiting a 100% specificity in distinguishing between benign and malignant mesothelial proliferations [52, 53], making it a valuable rule in test.

4. Staging

Staging helps classify the cancer based on the size of the tumor, its spread to nearby tissues and lymph nodes, as well as its potential metastasis to distant organs. This classification system provides valuable information that guides treatment decisions, such as whether surgery is a viable option, the potential benefits of chemotherapy or radiation therapy, and the overall prognosis for the patient. Historically, two staging systems were used for MPM following which the currently used TNM staging came into existence.

4.1 Butchart staging

Developed in 1976, the Butchart System consisting of four stages stands as the oldest formal staging system for mesothelioma and is exclusively utilized for staging pleural mesothelioma. This system relies solely on the location of the primary tumor mass to determine the stage and does not take into account factors such as tumor size or the overall extent of cancer present. This system had its limitations as the observations were based of a small study consisting of only 29 patients [54] and its ability for survival prediction is further limited by lack of inclusion of lymph node and chest wall involvement. The staging is described in **Table 3**.

4.2 Brigham Staging

Dr. David Sugarbaker of Boston's Brigham and Women's Hospital and colleagues introduced a staging system for malignant mesothelioma in 1993 [55], which was later revised in 1998. The system is based on two key factors: the operability of the mesothelioma through surgery and the involvement of lymph nodes. Derived from an analysis of 52 patients, It comprises of four stages as shown in **Table 3**.

4.3 TNM staging

In 1994, the International Mesothelioma Interest Group (IMIG) published the initial widely recognized tumor, node, and metastasis (TNM) classification for MPM [56]. This classification emerged from a consensus meeting held in June 1994 during the Seventh World Conference of the International Association for the Study of Lung Cancer (IASLC).

This has been the most widely used staging system and has been adopted by multiple societies like the International Union Against Cancer (UICC), the American Joint Committee on Cancer (AJCC), and the European Society for Radiotherapy and

Stage	Butchart Staging	Brigham Staging
1	Tumor confined to the parietal pleura	Tumor confined to the capsule of the parietal pleura, including ipsilateral pleura, lung, pericardium and diaphragm, or chest wall disease. Tumor is resectable
2	Invasion of the chest wall, esophagus, heart or contralateral pleura, with or without thoracic lymph node involvement	All Stage 1 disease with positive intrathoracic lymph nodes. Tumor is resectable
3	Invasion into diaphragm or extrathoracic lymph nodes	Local extension of disease into the chest wall or mediastinum, heart or through diaphragm into peritoneum, with or without extrathoracic or contralateral lymph node involvement. Tumor is unresectable
4	Distant extrathoracic metastatic disease	Distant extrathoracic metastatic disease. Tumor is unresectable

Table 3.
Butchart & Brigham Staging.

Oncology (ESTRO), among others. The latest version is the eighth TNM classification for MPM which was published in 2018.

As any of the other TNM classifications, the T descriptors (T1, T2, T3, and T4) define the local extent of the primary tumor. The N descriptors (N0, N1, N2, and N3) define nodal involvement and M represents evidence of metastasis.

Based on the TNM classification a staging system for this tumor was derived; stage I to IV. Some of the revisions of the latest version of the TNM classification for MPM includes removal of the N3 category and only M1 involvement is considered stage IV. Readers interested in detailed description are directed to review the eighth TNM classification for malignant pleural mesothelioma published in the journal of Translational Lung Cancer Research [57].

5. Treatment

Multimodality treatment is the foundation of therapy for MPM. Surgical therapy is a valued part of this approach.

5.1 Surgical

Surgical management for MPM is a part of a multimodal approach, which also includes chemotherapy and/or radiation therapy. The choice of surgery and overall management depends on factors such as the stage of the disease, the patient's overall health status, and potential for improved quality of life.

Patient selection for surgery is a critical step in the preoperative process. There are no absolute contraindications for surgery with respect to any comorbid condition.

Components of assessment include:

1. Functional status: understanding the patient's daily activity levels and physical capabilities is essential in predicting postoperative recovery and potential complications. Patient's functional status is generally assessed by ECOG performance scale [58].

2. Cardiac assessment: this is vital to determine the risk of cardiac complications during the peri-operative period. The revised cardiac risk index (RCRI) is typically used for cardiac assessments, identifying patients who need further cardiac evaluation due to high risk of complications [59]. Echocardiograms are conducted to exclude pulmonary hypertension.

3. Pulmonary function assessment: this testing is crucial, considering that thoracic surgery may impact respiratory function and help to identify patients with pre-existing pulmonary conditions. Preoperative pulmonary function tests are essential. Although there are no specific criterial regarding MPM, criteria for pneumonectomy in lung cancer includes a forced expiratory volume (FEV_1) > 2 L and diffusing capacity for carbon monoxide (DLCO) > 80%. If FEV_1 and DLCO fall below 80%, additional testing is mandated [60].

Considerations regarding surgical role include:

1. The surgical management of MPM demands careful preoperative staging with imaging and proper selection of patients based in performance status and cardiopulmonary reserve to evaluate those patients candidates for extra pleural pneumonectomy (EPP).

2. Aim for surgery is cytoreductive. Goal of surgical resection is macroscopic resection as this a diffusely growing tumor [61].

3. Results of isolated surgical therapy are poor and a multimodal approach with chemotherapy and/or radiation is necessary.

4. Type of surgery depends on factors such as the extent of disease, overall health of the patient, surgical risk, and potential for improved quality of life.

5. All patients with the diagnosis of MPM should be initially evaluated in a multidisciplinary setting, including medical and radiation oncology, and surgery.

6. Histological subtype by biopsy should precede therapy [61].

Procedures typically fall under one of two categories—aggressive surgery or palliative measures. Advanced stages of the disease (Stages II, III, and IV) often necessitate symptomatic treatment, which can include drainage of effusions or other measures to improve comfort and quality of life.

5.1.1 Aggressive surgery

While more extensive, aims at maximal removal of the disease. Median survival after the most radical surgery EPP is 18 months with a median survival of 14% at 5 years [62]. There are two major types of surgery used in the treatment of malignant mesothelioma.

5.1.1.1 Pleurectomy/decortication (P/D)

This is a lung-sparing surgery that involves removal of the pleura (the lining of the lung and chest wall) and any other visible tumor masses. This is often performed when the disease is more localized and the patient is otherwise in good health. This procedure can help to improve symptoms such as shortness of breath and chest pain. Subsequent to the surgical intervention, adjuvant therapies like radiation therapy, chemotherapy, and targeted therapy may serve a role in enhancing prognosis and managing the disease.

5.1.1.2 Extra pleural pneumonectomy

EPP involves the removal of the diseased lung, part of the pericardium, the diaphragm, and the parietal pleura. While this procedure can provide a more substantial disease reduction, it also comes with significantly more risk and potential for complications.

The choice between these procedures often depends on numerous factors such as the extent of disease, overall health of the patient, surgical risk, and potential for improved quality of life. However, it is crucial to factor the significant morbidity associated with these procedures. Patient selection is the key to successful outcomes and a multidisciplinary team often determines the optimal approach. In cases where the disease progression is advanced and cure is not feasible, the focus shifts towards palliative care, prioritizing the management of symptoms and improving the patient's quality of life.

Although there is controversy as to which procedure is better, lung sparing macroscopic resection was associated with comparable long-term outcomes with lower perioperative mortality [63]. P/D is associated with better long term survival for resectable MPM however post operative complications were higher in this group [64].

In a feasibility study on mesothelioma patients treated with standard care, those randomized to surgery and radiotherapy had a median survival of 14.4 months, contrasted with 19.5 months in the observation-only group [65]. However, due to a high dropout rate, the study lacked sufficient power. The forthcoming MARS 2 study is expected to provide more definitive insights [66].

5.1.2 Palliative surgery

When MPM is advanced and curative intent is not an option, surgery is helpful is symptom control and palliation. Pleural drainage reduces volume of effusion, dyspnea and cough in patients with trapped lung. Therapeutic options depend on patients' overall clinical status, ability to tolerate general anesthesia and presence of trapped lung. In high-risk patients, talc slurry under local anesthesia is an option, where as in patients who can tolerate general anesthesia, thoracoscopy with talc insufflation is an option as the procedure can be performed under direct vision [67]. A randomized control trial (RCT) compared VATS pleurodesis versus talc pleurodesis showed that talc pleurodesis might be preferable considering improved overall survival, fewer complications and shorter length of stay [68]. However, this included all patients with suspected malignant mesothelioma who had a pleural effusion and excluded patients with who has previous attempted pleurodesis and previous primary treatment for mesothelioma. VATS pleurodesis or partial pleurectomy (PP) is effective in management of recurrent effusions and entrapped lung.

As always, a comprehensive personalized discussion with the patient and a multidisciplinary team regarding treatment is paramount (**Table 4**).

Recommendations regarding surgical therapy as per ESMO clinical practice guidelines [25]*
1. Surgery: primarily advised for diagnosis, staging, and palliative purposes
2. Pleurodesis: talc poudrage via thoracostomy is the recommended procedure
3. Treatment in selected MPM patients: macroscopic resection, often combined with other treatments, is best performed at specialized, experienced centers
4. Surgical preference: Extended Pleurectomy and Decortication (EPD) is preferred over Extrapleural Pneumonectomy (EPP)

**Readers are encouraged to refer to the detailed recommendations. The table summarizes key features.*

Table 4.
Recommendations regarding surgical therapy.

5.2 Chemotherapy

Chemotherapy for MPM is used as a part of a multimodal treatment approach that may also include surgery and radiation therapy. It can be utilized in the neoadjuvant setting, adjuvant setting, in addition to palliative care. The aim is to reduce tumor volumes, improve symptom control, and enhance patient survival. Systemic therapy is based on staging and whether the disease is resectable or not (**Table 5**).

5.2.1 Resectable disease

In patients with resectable disease, standard practice consists of 4 cycles of neoadjuvant or adjuvant cisplatin-pemetrexed therapy. Bevacizumab is not recommended because of the high risk of bleeding during surgical resection.

5.2.2 Unresectable disease

The most common regimen for MPM is a combination of cisplatin and pemetrexed. Vogelzang et al. randomized 448 patients to cisplatin monotherapy vs. cisplatin- pemetrexed doublet therapy. This combination demonstrated an increased

Therapeutic options	**Pharmacologic group**	**Agents used**
First line agents	Alkylating agents	Cisplatin
	plus	
	Cytotoxic agents	Pemetrexed
	Nucleoside analogue	Gemcitabine
	plus	
	Alkylating agents	Cisplatin, carboplatin, oxaliplatin
Immunotherapy	Anti-Programmed Death-1 (PD-1) Antibody	Pembrolizumab, nivolumab ipilimumab
	Antiangiogenic therapy	Bevacizumab, sorafenib, sunitinib, cediranib, dovitinib

Table 5.
Chemotherapy/immunotherapy options for patients with MPM.

survival benefit compared to cisplatin alone in studies. Doublet therapy showed improved median survival 12.8 vs. 9 months, longer median time for disease progression (5.7 vs. 3.9 months) with a higher response rates (41.3% vs. 16.7%). Hematological toxicity (neutropenia) was higher in doublet arm and addition of folic acid and vitamin B12 resulted in significant reduction [69].

Gemcitabine, when combined with a platinum compound like cisplatin, carboplatin, or oxaliplatin, has undergone extensive testing in numerous phase II studies, showing variable response rates with acceptable toxicity levels [70–72]. Arrieta et al. [52] highlighted its efficacy, safety, and cost-effectiveness, particularly noting that Gemcitabine plus cisplatin is a viable and safe treatment for patients with unresectable MPM [47]. Carboplatin is an alternative when cisplatin is unsuitable.

In the refractory or second-line setting, agents such as gemcitabine or vinorelbine can be considered. It is important to consider patient's performance status, tumor histology, prior treatments, and side-effect profiles before deciding treatment. Chemotherapeutic agents have associated side effects, which include nausea, fatigue, neutropenia, and kidney toxicity.

5.3 Immunotherapy

5.3.1 Anti-Programmed Death-1 (PD-1) antibody

For patients with PDL-1 positive status, Pembrolizumab therapy is recommended. Specifically, in patients with previously treated PDL-1 positive malignant mesothelioma (MM), characterized by expression in 1% or more tumor cells, Pembrolizumab treatment up to 2 years, or until confirmed progression or unacceptable toxicity, demonstrated a 20% objective response rate, 72% disease control, and a median overall survival (OS) of 18 months [73].

The FDA approved Nivolumab plus Ipilimumab as a first-line treatment for adult patients with unresectable MPM, citing significant and clinically meaningful improvements in overall survival compared to standard-of-care chemotherapy [74]. Conversely, Pembrolizumab is not recommended as a stand-alone treatment for advanced, pretreated MPM [75].

5.3.2 Antiangiogenic therapy

Angiogenesis plays a crucial role in the development of malignant mesothelioma (MM). Bevacizumab, an angiogenesis inhibitor, has been investigated as a potential treatment option. The Mesothelioma Avastin Cisplatin Pemetrexed Study evaluated the impact of adding Bevacizumab to a first-line treatment regimen of cisplatin and pemetrexed for advanced MPM. This addition significantly enhanced overall survival in MPM patients, albeit with anticipated, manageable toxic effects [76].

Other anti-angiogenic therapies, including Sorafenib, Sunitinib, Cediranib, and Dovitinib, have not shown promising results in treating Malignant Pleural Mesothelioma (MPM) [77–80]. Currently, there is no consensus on treatment for patients who progress after cisplatin-based chemotherapy. Available options range from single-agent or combination immunotherapy, platinum-doublet immunotherapy, to Bevacizumab with Pemetrexed and Cisplatin therapy, depending on local expertise.

Ongoing advances in understanding MPM's pathogenesis aim to optimize traditional treatments like chemotherapy and integrate new molecular targeted therapies into treatment protocols for this aggressive disease (**Table 6**).

Recommendations regarding systemic therapy as per ESMO clinical practice guidelines [25]*
First line therapy for malignant pleural mesothelioma (MPM) 1. Pemetrexed and platinum-based chemotherapy • Standard: pemetrexed combined with cisplatin. • Alternative: pemetrexed with carboplatin. • Addition: vitamin supplementation. 2. Bevacizumab combination therapy 3. Composition: bevacizumab combined with platinum (cisplatin or carboplatin) and pemetrexed.
Recommendations for Unresectable MPM Nivolumab Plus Ipilimumab Criteria: recommended for unresectable MPM regardless of histologies or PD-L1 status.
Maintenance therapy in non-progressive MPM 1. Gemcitabine maintenance Guideline: not routinely recommended in non-progressive MPM. 2. Pemetrexed maintenance Guideline: not routinely recommended after first-line therapy in non-progressive MPM.
**Readers are encouraged to refer to the detailed recommendations. The table summarizes key features.*

Table 6.
Systemic therapy as per ESMO guidelines.

5.3.3 Systemic therapy for second line and beyond

5.3.3.1 Options for systemic therapy for second line and beyond

Treatment options for immunotherapy-naïve malignant pleural mesothelioma (MPM) patients

1. Immunotherapy options
   - Pembrolizumab: an option for immunotherapy-naïve patients.
   - Nivolumab: demonstrated superiority over best supportive care
   - Nivolumab-Ipilimumab combination: considered as a third or fourth line of treatment.
2. Subsequent treatment strategies

   a. Reintroduction of chemotherapy
   - Options include platinum-pemetrexed or pemetrexed chemotherapy.

   b. Gemcitabine-ramucirumab combination
   - An alternative treatment option.

   c. Post-failure strategy
   - No routine third-line therapy recommended after failure of initial options.

d. Clinical trial participation

- Considered as a last resort for treatment exploration.

5.3.3.2 Future directions

A wide array of clinical trials is ongoing, targeting various aspects of MPM pathophysiology. While many trials have been completed, others are actively recruiting participants. These trials are expected to provide critical insights and potentially more effective therapeutic options for MPM patients and results may significantly enhance our understanding and management of MPM.

5.3.3.3 Recommended reading for future perspectives

Pezzoli et al.'s Special Article: Titled "A Glimpse in the Future of Malignant Mesothelioma Treatment," this article offers valuable insights into prospective developments in MPM treatment [81].

5.4 Radiation therapy

For malignant mesothelioma, radiation therapy (RT) has been explored as both a primary and ancillary intervention. This can be delivered in the adjuvant, neoadjuvant and palliative settings.

In terms of primary intervention, external beam radiotherapy (EBRT) may be employed for curative intent, palliative pain relief, or control of symptoms like dyspnea. Pros and cons are, however, at balance. While EBRT has failed to show definitive overall survival benefit, recent advances such as Intensity-Modulated Radiation Therapy (IMRT) have demonstrated potential by enabling a more targeted irradiation and reducing toxicity to surrounding organs.

Adjuvant radiotherapy following surgical procedures [like extra pleural pneumonectomy (EPP) or pleurectomy/decortication (P/D)] has been another domain of interest. Traditionally, prophylactic irradiation of procedure sites was used to prevent tract seeding, based on earlier studies [82, 83]. Subsequent trials have revealed no benefit of prophylactic radiotherapy to diagnostic or therapeutic procedure tracks [84, 85].

There is also the strategy of trimodality therapy—combining surgery, chemotherapy, and RT. Stahel et al. reported that high-dose hemi-thoracic radiotherapy after neoadjuvant chemotherapy and EPP in patients with MPM. The study observed an increase in relapse-free survival from 7.6 months in patients who did not receive RT to 9.4 months in the group that underwent RT post-chemotherapy and EPP [86]. Despite the demonstrated safety, the ideal criteria for selecting patients who would most benefit from this aggressive trimodal therapy (surgery, chemotherapy, and RT) are not well-defined [87]. The findings underscore the need for further research to establish clear guidelines for selecting patients for trimodal therapy, aiming to maximize benefits while minimizing risks. Existing evidence on trimodal therapy is equivocal and it may be best suited for select patients with good performance status and limited disease spread.

5.4.1 Palliative RT

Radiotherapy can be used in palliation of pain, SVC syndrome, metastatic lesions and obstructive symptoms. Mcleod et al. assessed the role of RT for the treatment of pain in

Recommendations regarding radiation therapy as per ESMO clinical practice guidelines [25]*
1. *Palliation of pain due to local infiltration* RT serves as a treatment option for alleviating pain associated with local tumor infiltration.
2. *Discontinued use of prophylactic RT* Prophylactic radiotherapy to tracts post-diagnostic or therapeutic pleural procedures is no longer recommended for preventing chest wall metastases.
3. *RT in adjuvant setting post-resection* Consideration of RT as an adjuvant therapy is viable following complete tumor resection.
4. *Minimizing toxicity in postoperative RT* Emphasis on avoiding toxicity to adjacent organs at risk when applying postoperative radiotherapy.
**Readers are encouraged to refer to the detailed recommendations. The table above summarizes key features.*

Table 7.
Recommendations for radiation therapy.

MPM. Complete case analysis of the 30 patients assessable at week 5, revealed improvement of pain in 47% of patients alive at week 5 [88]. SYSTEMS-2 is a randomized study of RT dose escalation for pain control in 112 patients with malignant pleural mesothelioma (MPM). Standard palliative (20 Gy/5#) or dose escalated treatment (36 Gy/6#) will be delivered using advanced radiotherapy techniques and pain responses will be compared at week 5. Data will guide optimal palliative radiotherapy in MPM [89].

Radiation therapy is an evolving field in mesothelioma management. As clinical experience with newer radiation modalities grows, radiation therapy may provide benefit for these patients (**Table 7**).

6. Prognosis

The prognosis for MPM depends on several factors, including age, gender, stage at diagnosis, patient's performance status, and the effectiveness of treatment [8, 90–92].

Stage: The stage of the disease at the time of diagnosis is a critical factor in determining prognosis. Mesothelioma is typically staged from I to IV, with stage I being localized and easier to treat, while stage IV indicates advanced disease that has spread to distant organs. Early-stage mesothelioma generally has a better prognosis than advanced-stage disease.

Treatment: Mesothelioma treatment options may include surgery, chemotherapy, RT and immunotherapy. The effectiveness of treatment and the patient's response to it can significantly affect prognosis. Some patients may undergo multimodal treatment approaches.

Age and overall health: A patient's age and overall health play a role in determining their prognosis. Younger, healthier individuals may have a better chance of tolerating aggressive treatments and achieving longer-term survival.

Mesothelioma cell type: Of three primary cell types of mesothelioma: epithelioid, sarcomatoid, and biphasic (a combination of both), epithelioid mesothelioma generally has a better prognosis than the other two cell types [93, 94].

Genetic and molecular factors: Recent research has identified specific genetic mutations and molecular markers associated with mesothelioma. Recently GOLT1B and MAD2L1 expression was reported as the best predictor of survival [95]. Three promising emerging therapeutic targets include STAT3, KDM4A, heparanase [96].

6.1 Prognostic scoring systems

6.1.1 Multimodality prognostic score

Multimodality prognostic score (MMPS) was reported by Opiz et al. [97]. These include

1. Tumor volume pretreatment greater than 500 ml

2. Non-epithelioid histology

3. Serum C-reactive protein value greater than 30 mg/L

4. Progression after induction chemotherapy assessed by modified Response Evaluation Criteria in Solid Tumors (RECIST 1.1 are standardized criteria that can be used at different time points to classify response into the categories of complete response, partial response, stable disease, or disease progression).

The score identified group of patient not benefitting from multimodality treatment (Score ≤ 2 vs. ≥2) 21 (15–28) vs. 4 (3–5) months P ≤ 0.0005). The MMPS (using three or four variables) showed that patients with score 0 had the longest overall survival compared with those with a score of 3 or higher.

In patients with MPM, pretreatment serum albumin level is a marker of prognostic significance [98]. In a subsequent publication, adding albumin to the initial MMPS score showed improved performance in comparison to the original score [99]. Using a classification and regression tree (CART) model Harris et all reported the group of patients with no weight loss, hemoglobin >15 g/L and serum albumin >4.3 g/L at time of referral to the surgical center has the best survival [100]. Several gene markers have looked at prognosis in patients with MM [17, 101, 102]. In newly diagnosed patients with MPM, use of pretreatment parameters may help to prognosticate outcomes after surgery and also enhance stratification on clinical trials [103].

6.1.2 Cancer and leukemia group B (CALGB) index

CALBG index was developed retrospectively using clinical characteristics of 337 patients [7]. Six prognostic groups can be determined with median survival ranging between 29.9 months in the most favorable group to 1.8 for the least favorable one. Pleural disease involvement, LDH level > 500 lUlL, poor PS, chest pain, platelet count >400,000/f.LL, nonepitheloid histology, and increasing age older than 75 years independently predict poorer survival. These findings were confirmed by a subsequent study [104].

6.1.3 European Organization for Research and Treatment of Cancer experience (EORTC) index

ORTC index was also developed retrospectively during a 9-year period from October 1984 to October 1993. 204 eligible adult patients with MPM were entered into five consecutive prospective EORTC phase II clinical trials designed to assess the efficacy of various anticancer drugs (mitoxantrone, epidoxorubicin, etoposide, and paclitaxel) [6]. Patients with poor functional status, elevated WBC counts, mesothelioma as a probable/possible diagnosis, male gender and sarcomatous histological subtype had a poor prognosis.

7. Conclusion

It is important to note that MPM is often diagnosed at an advanced stage, which can make it challenging to treat effectively. As a result, the overall prognosis for mesothelioma is generally poor, with a median survival of around 12–21 months for pleural mesothelioma. However, advancements in treatment options, such as immunotherapy and targeted therapies, have provided some hope for improved outcomes, particularly for those with earlier-stage disease or specific molecular markers. Early suspicion and aggressive diagnosis is recommended to improve outcomes.

Conflict of interest

The authors declare no conflict of interest.

Author details

Nishant Allena*, Sindhaghatta Venkatram and Gilda Diaz-Fuentes
Division of Pulmonary Medicine and Critical Care, BronxCare Health System, New York, United States

*Address all correspondence to: nishantallena24@gmail.com

References

[1] Robinson BW, Lake RA. Advances in malignant mesothelioma. The New England Journal of Medicine. 2005;**353**(15):1591-1603

[2] McDonald JC, McDonald AD. The epidemiology of mesothelioma in historical context. The European Respiratory Journal. 1996;**9**(9):1932-1942

[3] Franko A, Dolzan V, Kovac V, Arneric N, Dodic-Fikfak M. Soluble mesothelin-related peptides levels in patients with malignant mesothelioma. Disease Markers. 2012;**32**(2):123-131

[4] Delgermaa V, Takahashi K, Park EK, Le GV, Hara T, Sorahan T. Global mesothelioma deaths reported to the World Health Organization between 1994 and 2008. Bulletin of the World Health Organization. 2011;**89**(10):716-724, 24A-24C

[5] Driscoll T, Nelson DI, Steenland K, Leigh J, Concha-Barrientos M, Fingerhut M, et al. The global burden of disease due to occupational carcinogens. American Journal of Industrial Medicine. 2005;**48**(6):419-431

[6] Curran D, Sahmoud T, Therasse P, van Meerbeeck J, Postmus PE, Giaccone G. Prognostic factors in patients with pleural mesothelioma: The European Organization for Research and Treatment of Cancer experience. Journal of Clinical Oncology. 1998;**16**(1):145-152

[7] Herndon JE, Green MR, Chahinian AP, Corson JM, Suzuki Y, Vogelzang NJ. Factors predictive of survival among 337 patients with mesothelioma treated between 1984 and 1994 by the cancer and leukemia group B. Chest. 1998;**113**(3):723-731

[8] Rahouma M, Aziz H, Ghaly G, Kamel M, Loai I, Mohamed A. Survival in good performance malignant pleural mesothelioma patients; prognostic factors and predictors of response. Asian Pacific Journal of Cancer Prevention. 2017;**18**(8):2073-2078

[9] Baas P, Fennell D, Kerr KM, Van Schil PE, Haas RL, Peters S, et al. Malignant pleural mesothelioma: ESMO clinical practice guidelines for diagnosis, treatment and follow-up. Annals of Oncology. 2015;**26**(Suppl 5):v31-v39

[10] Tsao AS, Wistuba I, Roth JA, Kindler HL. Malignant pleural mesothelioma. Journal of Clinical Oncology. 2009;**27**(12):2081-2090

[11] Carbone M, Ferris LK, Baumann F, Napolitano A, Lum CA, Flores EG, et al. BAP1 cancer syndrome: Malignant mesothelioma, uveal and cutaneous melanoma, and MBAITs. Journal of Translational Medicine. 2012;**10**:179

[12] Hillerdal G. Pleural plaques and risk for bronchial carcinoma and mesothelioma. A prospective study. Chest. 1994;**105**(1):144-150

[13] Pairon JC, Laurent F, Rinaldo M, Clin B, Andujar P, Ameille J, et al. Pleural plaques and the risk of pleural mesothelioma. Journal of the National Cancer Institute. 2013;**105**(4):293-301

[14] Reid A, de Klerk N, Ambrosini G, Olsen N, Pang SC, Musk AW. The additional risk of malignant mesothelioma in former workers and residents of Wittenoom with benign pleural disease or asbestosis. Occupational and Environmental Medicine. 2005;**62**(10):665-669

[15] Chew SH, Toyokuni S. Malignant mesothelioma as an oxidative stress-induced cancer: An update. Free Radical Biology & Medicine. 2015;**86**:166-178

[16] Liu G, Cheresh P, Kamp DW. Molecular basis of asbestos-induced lung disease. Annual Review of Pathology. 2013;**8**:161-187

[17] Bueno R, Stawiski EW, Goldstein LD, Durinck S, De Rienzo A, Modrusan Z, et al. Comprehensive genomic analysis of malignant pleural mesothelioma identifies recurrent mutations, gene fusions and splicing alterations. Nature Genetics. 2016;**48**(4):407-416

[18] Carbone M, Yang H. Mesothelioma: Recent highlights. Annals of Translational Medicine. 2017;**5**(11):238

[19] Huang SX, Jaurand MC, Kamp DW, Whysner J, Hei TK. Role of mutagenicity in asbestos fiber-induced carcinogenicity and other diseases. Journal of Toxicology and Environmental Health. Part B, Critical Reviews. 2011;**14**(1-4):179-245

[20] Bibby AC, Tsim S, Kanellakis N, Ball H, Talbot DC, Blyth KG, et al. Malignant pleural mesothelioma: An update on investigation, diagnosis and treatment. European Respiratory Review. 2016;**25**(142):472-486

[21] Rusch VW. Diagnosis and treatment of pleural mesothelioma. Seminars in Surgical Oncology. 1990;**6**(5):279-285

[22] Xie XF, Huang Y, Guo JH, Zhang W, Hou LK, Wu CY, et al. Often misdiagnosed primary pleural epithelioid hemangioendothelioma: A clinicopathological analysis of five cases. Zhonghua Bing Li Xue Za Zhi. 2020;**49**(12):1288-1293

[23] Stewart DJ, Edwards JG, Smythe WR, Waller DA, O'Byrne KJ. Malignant pleural mesothelioma—An update. International Journal of Occupational and Environmental Health. 2004;**10**(1):26-39

[24] Devroede GJ, Tirol AF. Giant pleural mesothelioma associated with hypoglycemia and hyperthyroidism. American Journal of Surgery. 1968;**116**(1):130-134

[25] Popat S, Baas P, Faivre-Finn C, Girard N, Nicholson AG, Nowak AK, et al. Malignant pleural mesothelioma: ESMO clinical practice guidelines for diagnosis, treatment and follow-up(☆). Annals of Oncology. 2022;**33**(2):129-142

[26] Sneddon S, Dick I, Lee YCG, Musk AWB, Patch AM, Pearson JV, et al. Malignant cells from pleural fluids in malignant mesothelioma patients reveal novel mutations. Lung Cancer. 2018;**119**:64-70

[27] Bianco A, Valente T, De Rimini ML, Sica G, Fiorelli A. Clinical diagnosis of malignant pleural mesothelioma. Journal of Thoracic Disease. 2018;**10**(Suppl 2):S253-SS61

[28] Goricar K, Kovac V, Franko A, Dodic-Fikfak M, Dolzan V. Serum survivin levels and outcome of chemotherapy in patients with malignant mesothelioma. Disease Markers. 2015;**2015**:316739

[29] Pass HI, Levin SM, Harbut MR, Melamed J, Chiriboga L, Donington J, et al. Fibulin-3 as a blood and effusion biomarker for pleural mesothelioma. The New England Journal of Medicine. 2012;**367**(15):1417-1427

[30] Scherpereel A, Grigoriu B, Conti M, Gey T, Gregoire M, Copin MC, et al. Soluble mesothelin-related peptides in the diagnosis of malignant pleural mesothelioma. American Journal of

Respiratory and Critical Care Medicine. 2006;**173**(10):1155-1160

[31] Brusselmans L, Arnouts L, Millevert C, Vandersnickt J, van Meerbeeck JP, Lamote K. Breath analysis as a diagnostic and screening tool for malignant pleural mesothelioma: A systematic review. Translational Lung Cancer Research. 2018;**7**(5):520-536

[32] Testa JR, Cheung M, Pei J, Below JE, Tan Y, Sementino E, et al. Germline BAP1 mutations predispose to malignant mesothelioma. Nature Genetics. 2011;**43**(10):1022-1025

[33] Tamer Dogan O, Salk I, Tas F, Epozturk K, Gumus C, Akkurt I, et al. Thoracic computed tomography findings in malignant mesothelioma. Iranian Journal of Radiology. 2012;**9**(4):209-211

[34] Vivoda Tomšič M, Bisdas S, Kovač V, Serša I, Šurlan PK. Dynamic contrast-enhanced MRI of malignant pleural mesothelioma: A comparative study of pharmacokinetic models and correlation with mRECIST criteria. Cancer Imaging. 2019;**19**(1):10

[35] Weber MA, Bock M, Plathow C, Wasser K, Fink C, Zuna I, et al. Asbestos-related pleural disease: Value of dedicated magnetic resonance imaging techniques. Investigative Radiology. 2004;**39**(9):554-564

[36] Volpi F, D'Amore CA, Colligiani L, Milazzo A, Cavaliere S, De Liperi A, et al. The use of chest magnetic resonance imaging in malignant pleural mesothelioma diagnosis. Diagnostics (Basel). 2022;**12**(3):70

[37] Patel AM, Berger I, Wileyto EP, Khalid U, Torigian DA, Nachiappan AC, et al. The value of delayed phase enhanced imaging in malignant pleural mesothelioma. Journal of Thoracic Disease. 2017;**9**(8):2344-2349

[38] Taralli S, Giancipoli RG, Caldarella C, Scolozzi V, Ricciardi S, Cardillo G, et al. The prognostic value of (18)F-FDG PET imaging at staging in patients with malignant pleural mesothelioma: A literature review. Journal of Clinical Medicine. 2021;**11**(1):33

[39] Wen W, Xu D, Piao Y, Li X. Prognostic value of maximum standard uptake value, metabolic tumour volume, and total lesion glycolysis of 18F-FDG PET/CT in patients with malignant pleural mesothelioma: A systematic review and meta-analysis. Cancer Cell International. 2022;**22**(1):60

[40] Hiriart E, Deepe R, Wessels A. Mesothelium and malignant mesothelioma. Journal of Developmental Biology. 2019;**7**(2)

[41] Hollevoet K, Reitsma JB, Creaney J, Grigoriu BD, Robinson BW, Scherpereel A, et al. Serum mesothelin for diagnosing malignant pleural mesothelioma: An individual patient data meta-analysis. Journal of Clinical Oncology. 2012;**30**(13):1541-1549

[42] Creaney J, Christansen H, Lake R, Musk AB, de Klerk N, Robinson BW. Soluble mesothelin related protein in mesothelioma. Journal of Thoracic Oncology. 2006;**1**(2):172-174

[43] Pass HI, Lott D, Lonardo F, Harbut M, Liu Z, Tang N, et al. Asbestos exposure, pleural mesothelioma, and serum osteopontin levels. The New England Journal of Medicine. 2005;**353**(15):1564-1573

[44] Napolitano A, Antoine DJ, Pellegrini L, Baumann F, Pagano I, Pastorino S, et al. HMGB1 and its hyperacetylated isoform are sensitive

and specific serum biomarkers to detect asbestos exposure and to identify mesothelioma patients. Clinical Cancer Research. 2016;**22**(12):3087-3096

[45] Bielsa S, Panadés MJ, Egido R, Rue M, Salud A, Matías-Guiu X, et al. Accuracy of pleural fluid cytology in malignant effusions. Anales de Medicina Interna. 2008;**25**(4):173-177

[46] Husain AN, Colby T, Ordonez N, Krausz T, Attanoos R, Beasley MB, et al. Guidelines for pathologic diagnosis of malignant mesothelioma: 2012 update of the consensus statement from the International Mesothelioma Interest Group. Archives of Pathology & Laboratory Medicine. 2013;**137**(5):647-667

[47] Lang-Lazdunski L. Surgery for malignant pleural mesothelioma: Why, when and what? Lung Cancer. 2014;**84**(2):103-109

[48] Scherpereel A, Opitz I, Berghmans T, Psallidas I, Glatzer M, Rigau D, et al. ERS/ESTS/EACTS/ESTRO guidelines for the management of malignant pleural mesothelioma. The European Respiratory Journal. 2020;**55**(6):1900953

[49] Alì G, Bruno R, Fontanini G. The pathological and molecular diagnosis of malignant pleural mesothelioma: A literature review. Journal of Thoracic Disease. 2018;**10**(Suppl 2):S276-Ss84

[50] Klebe S, Mahar A, Henderson DW, Roggli VL. Malignant mesothelioma with heterologous elements: Clinicopathological correlation of 27 cases and literature review. Modern Pathology. 2008;**21**(9):1084-1094

[51] Travis WD, Brambilla E, Burke AP, Marx A, Nicholson AG. Introduction to the 2015 World Health Organization classification of tumors of the lung, pleura, thymus, and heart. Journal of Thoracic Oncology. 2015;**10**(9):1240-1242

[52] Arrieta O, Munoz-Montano W, Muniz-Hernandez S, Campos S, Catalan R, Soto-Molina H, et al. Efficacy, safety, and cost-minimization analysis of continuous infusion of low-dose gemcitabine plus cisplatin in patients with unresectable malignant pleural mesothelioma. Frontiers in Oncology. 2021;**11**:641975

[53] Cigognetti M, Lonardi S, Fisogni S, Balzarini P, Pellegrini V, Tironi A, et al. BAP1 (BRCA1-associated protein 1) is a highly specific marker for differentiating mesothelioma from reactive mesothelial proliferations. Modern Pathology. 2015;**28**(8):1043-1057

[54] Butchart EGGA. Pleural mesothelioma. Current Opinion in Oncology. 1990;**2**:352-358

[55] Sugarbaker DJ, Strauss GM, Lynch TJ, Richards W, Mentzer SJ, Lee TH, et al. Node status has prognostic significance in the multimodality therapy of diffuse, malignant mesothelioma. Journal of Clinical Oncology. 1993;**11**(6):1172-1178

[56] Rusch VW. A proposed new international TNM staging system for malignant pleural mesothelioma. From the International Mesothelioma Interest Group. Chest. 1995;**108**(4):1122-1128

[57] Berzenji L, Van Schil PE, Carp L. The eighth TNM classification for malignant pleural mesothelioma. Translational Lung Cancer Research. 2018;7(5):543-549

[58] Oken MM, Creech RH, Tormey DC, Horton J, Davis TE, McFadden ET, et al. Toxicity and response criteria of the Eastern Cooperative Oncology Group.

American Journal of Clinical Oncology. 1982;**5**(6):649-655

[59] Fleisher LA, Beckman JA, Brown KA, Calkins H, Chaikof EL, Fleischmann KE, et al. ACC/AHA 2007 guidelines on perioperative cardiovascular evaluation and care for noncardiac surgery: A report of the American College of Cardiology/American Heart Association Task Force on Practice Guidelines (Writing Committee to Revise the 2002 Guidelines on Perioperative Cardiovascular Evaluation for Noncardiac Surgery) developed in collaboration with the American Society of Echocardiography, American Society of Nuclear Cardiology, Heart Rhythm Society, Society of Cardiovascular Anesthesiologists, Society for Cardiovascular Angiography and Interventions, Society for Vascular Medicine and Biology, and Society for Vascular Surgery. Journal of the American College of Cardiology. 2007;**50**(17):e159-e241

[60] Roy PM. Preoperative pulmonary evaluation for lung resection. Journal of Anaesthesiology Clinical Pharmacology. 2018;**34**(3):296-300

[61] Rusch V, Baldini EH, Bueno R, De Perrot M, Flores R, Hasegawa S, et al. The role of surgical cytoreduction in the treatment of malignant pleural mesothelioma: Meeting summary of the international Mesothelioma Interest Group Congress, September 11-14, 2012, Boston, Mass. Journal of Thoracic and Cardiovascular Surgery. 2013;**145**(4):909-910

[62] Sugarbaker DJ, Richards WG, Bueno R. Extrapleural pneumonectomy in the treatment of epithelioid malignant pleural mesothelioma: Novel prognostic implications of combined N1 and N2 nodal involvement based on experience in 529 patients. Annals of Surgery. 2014;**260**(4):577-580; discussion 80-2.

[63] Zhou N, Rice DC, Tsao AS, Lee PP, Haymaker CL, Corsini EM, et al. Extrapleural pneumonectomy versus pleurectomy/decortication for malignant pleural mesothelioma. The Annals of Thoracic Surgery. 2022;**113**(1):200-208

[64] Danuzzo F, Maiorca S, Bonitta G, Nosotti M. Systematic review and meta-analysis of pleurectomy/decortication versus extrapleural pneumonectomy in the treatment of malignant pleural mesothelioma. Journal of Clinical Medicine. 2022;**11**(19):5544

[65] Treasure T, Lang-Lazdunski L, Waller D, Bliss JM, Tan C, Entwisle J, et al. Extra-pleural pneumonectomy versus no extra-pleural pneumonectomy for patients with malignant pleural mesothelioma: Clinical outcomes of the Mesothelioma and Radical Surgery (MARS) randomised feasibility study. The Lancet Oncology. 2011;**12**(8):763-772

[66] Lim E, Darlison L, Edwards J, Elliott D, Fennell DA, Popat S, et al. Mesothelioma and Radical Surgery 2 (MARS 2): Protocol for a multicentre randomised trial comparing (extended) pleurectomy decortication versus no (extended) pleurectomy decortication for patients with malignant pleural mesothelioma. BMJ Open. 2020;**10**(9):e038892

[67] Novello S, Pinto C, Torri V, Porcu L, Di Maio M, Tiseo M, et al. The third Italian consensus conference for malignant pleural mesothelioma: State of the art and recommendations. Critical Reviews in Oncology/Hematology. 2016;**104**:9-20

[68] Rintoul RC, Ritchie AJ, Edwards JG, Waller DA, Coonar AS, Bennett M, et al. Efficacy and cost of video-assisted thoracoscopic partial pleurectomy versus talc pleurodesis in patients with malignant pleural mesothelioma

(MesoVATS): An open-label, randomised, controlled trial. Lancet. 2014;**384**(9948):1118-1127

[69] Vogelzang NJ, Rusthoven JJ, Symanowski J, Denham C, Kaukel E, Ruffie P, et al. Phase III study of pemetrexed in combination with cisplatin versus cisplatin alone in patients with malignant pleural mesothelioma. Journal of Clinical Oncology. 2003;**21**(14):2636-2644

[70] Janne PA, Simon GR, Langer CJ, Taub RN, Dowlati A, Fidias P, et al. Phase II trial of pemetrexed and gemcitabine in chemotherapy-naive malignant pleural mesothelioma. Journal of Clinical Oncology. 2008;**26**(9):1465-1471

[71] Schutte W, Blankenburg T, Lauerwald K, Schreiber J, Bork I, Wollscgkaeger B, et al. A multicenter phase II study of gemcitabine and oxaliplatin for malignant pleural mesothelioma. Clinical Lung Cancer. 2003;**4**(5):294-297

[72] Favaretto AG, Aversa SM, Paccagnella A, Manzini Vde P, Palmisano V, Oniga F, et al. Gemcitabine combined with carboplatin in patients with malignant pleural mesothelioma: A multicentric phase II study. Cancer. 2003;**97**(11):2791-2797

[73] Alley EW, Lopez J, Santoro A, Morosky A, Saraf S, Piperdi B, et al. Clinical safety and activity of pembrolizumab in patients with malignant pleural mesothelioma (KEYNOTE-028): Preliminary results from a non-randomised, open-label, phase 1b trial. The Lancet Oncology. 2017;**18**(5):623-630

[74] Baas P, Scherpereel A, Nowak AK, Fujimoto N, Peters S, Tsao AS, et al. First-line nivolumab plus ipilimumab in unresectable malignant pleural mesothelioma (CheckMate 743): A multicentre, randomised, open-label, phase 3 trial. Lancet. 2021;**397**(10272):375-386

[75] Popat S, Curioni-Fontecedro A, Dafni U, Shah R, O'Brien M, Pope A, et al. A multicentre randomised phase III trial comparing pembrolizumab versus single-agent chemotherapy for advanced pre-treated malignant pleural mesothelioma: The European Thoracic Oncology Platform (ETOP 9-15) PROMISE-meso trial. Annals of Oncology. 2020;**31**(12):1734-1745

[76] Zalcman G, Mazieres J, Margery J, Greillier L, Audigier-Valette C, Moro-Sibilot D, et al. Bevacizumab for newly diagnosed pleural mesothelioma in the Mesothelioma Avastin Cisplatin Pemetrexed Study (MAPS): A randomised, controlled, open-label, phase 3 trial. Lancet. 2016;**387**(10026):1405-1414

[77] Papa S, Popat S, Shah R, Prevost AT, Lal R, McLennan B, et al. Phase 2 study of sorafenib in malignant mesothelioma previously treated with platinum-containing chemotherapy. Journal of Thoracic Oncology. 2013;**8**(6):783-787

[78] Laurie SA, Gupta A, Chu Q, Lee CW, Morzycki W, Feld R, et al. Brief report: A phase II study of sunitinib in malignant pleural mesothelioma. Tthe NCIC Clinical Trials Group. Journal of Thoracic Oncology. 2011;**6**(11):1950-1954

[79] Laurie SA, Hao D, Leighl NB, Goffin J, Khomani A, Gupta A, et al. A phase II trial of dovitinib in previously-treated advanced pleural mesothelioma: The Ontario Clinical Oncology Group. Lung Cancer. 2017;**104**:65-69

[80] Tsao AS, Miao J, Wistuba II, Vogelzang NJ, Heymach JV, Fossella FV, et al. Phase II trial of cediranib in combination

with cisplatin and pemetrexed in chemotherapy-naive patients with unresectable malignant pleural mesothelioma (SWOG S0905). Journal of Clinical Oncology. 2019;**37**(28):2537-2547

[81] Pezzicoli G, Rizzo M, Perrone M, Minei S, Mutti L, Porta C. A glimpse in the future of malignant mesothelioma treatment. Frontiers in Pharmacology. 2021;**12**:809337

[82] Froment MA, Frechette E, Dagnault A. Prophylactic irradiation of intervention sites in malignant pleural mesothelioma. Radiotherapy and Oncology. 2011;**101**(2):307-310

[83] Boutin C, Rey F, Viallat JR. Prevention of malignant seeding after invasive diagnostic procedures in patients with pleural mesothelioma. A randomized trial of local radiotherapy. Chest. 1995;**108**(3):754-758

[84] Clive AO, Taylor H, Dobson L, Wilson P, de Winton E, Panakis N, et al. Prophylactic radiotherapy for the prevention of procedure-tract metastases after surgical and large-bore pleural procedures in malignant pleural mesothelioma (SMART): A multicentre, open-label, phase 3, randomised controlled trial. The Lancet Oncology. 2016;**17**(8):1094-1104

[85] Bayman N, Appel W, Ashcroft L, Baldwin DR, Bates A, Darlison L, et al. Prophylactic irradiation of tracts in patients with malignant pleural mesothelioma: An open-label, multicenter, phase III randomized trial. Journal of Clinical Oncology. 2019;**37**(14):1200-1208

[86] Stahel RA, Riesterer O, Xyrafas A, Opitz I, Beyeler M, Ochsenbein A, et al. Neoadjuvant chemotherapy and extrapleural pneumonectomy of malignant pleural mesothelioma with or without hemithoracic radiotherapy (SAKK 17/04): A randomised, international, multicentre phase 2 trial. The Lancet Oncology. 2015;**16**(16):1651-1658

[87] Thieke C, Nicolay NH, Sterzing F, Hoffmann H, Roeder F, Safi S, et al. Long-term results in malignant pleural mesothelioma treated with neoadjuvant chemotherapy, extrapleural pneumonectomy and intensity-modulated radiotherapy. Radiation Oncology. 2015;**10**:267

[88] MacLeod N, Chalmers A, O'Rourke N, Moore K, Sheridan J, McMahon L, et al. Is radiotherapy useful for treating pain in mesothelioma?: A phase II trial. Journal of Thoracic Oncology. 2015;**10**(6):944-950

[89] Ashton M, O'Rourke N, Macleod N, Laird B, Stobo J, Kelly C, et al. SYSTEMS-2: A randomised phase II study of radiotherapy dose escalation for pain control in malignant pleural mesothelioma. Clinical and Translational Radiation Oncology. 2018;**8**:45-49

[90] Edwards JG, Abrams KR, Leverment JN, Spyt TJ, Waller DA, O'Byrne KJ. Prognostic factors for malignant mesothelioma in 142 patients: Validation of CALGB and EORTC prognostic scoring systems. Thorax. 2000;**55**(9):731-735

[91] Haber SE, Haber JM. Malignant mesothelioma: A clinical study of 238 cases. Industrial Health. 2011;**49**(2):166-172

[92] Shavelle R, Vavra-Musser K, Lee J, Brooks J. Life expectancy in pleural and peritoneal mesothelioma. Lung Cancer International. 2017;**2017**:2782590

[93] Alchami FS, Attanoos RL, Bamber AR. Myxoid variant epithelioid

pleural mesothelioma defines a favourable prognosis group: An analysis of 191 patients with pleural malignant mesothelioma. Journal of Clinical Pathology. 2017;**70**(2):179-182

[94] Kadota K, Suzuki K, Sima CS, Rusch VW, Adusumilli PS, Travis WD. Pleomorphic epithelioid diffuse malignant pleural mesothelioma: A clinicopathological review and conceptual proposal to reclassify as biphasic or sarcomatoid mesothelioma. Journal of Thoracic Oncology. 2011;**6**(5):896-904

[95] Shivarov V, Blazhev G, Yordanov A. A novel two-gene expression-based prognostic score in malignant pleural mesothelioma. Diagnostics (Basel). 2023;**13**(9):1661

[96] Lapidot M, Saladi SV, Salgia R, Sattler M. Novel therapeutic targets and immune dysfunction in malignant pleural mesothelioma. Frontiers in Pharmacology. 2021;**12**:806570

[97] Opitz I, Friess M, Kestenholz P, Schneiter D, Frauenfelder T, Nguyen-Kim TD, et al. A new prognostic score supporting treatment allocation for multimodality therapy for malignant pleural mesothelioma: A review of 12 years' experience. Journal of Thoracic Oncology. 2015;**10**(11):1634-1641

[98] Yao ZH, Tian GY, Yang SX, Wan YY, Kang YM, Liu QH, et al. Serum albumin as a significant prognostic factor in patients with malignant pleural mesothelioma. Tumour Biology. 2014;**35**(7):6839-6845

[99] Greb D, Hebeisen M, Matter A, Opitz I, Lauk O. Prospective validation and extension of the multimodality prognostic score for the treatment allocation of pleural mesothelioma patients. European Journal of Cardio-Thoracic Surgery. 2022;**62**(2)

[100] Harris EJA, Kao S, McCaughan B, Nakano T, Kondo N, Hyland R, et al. Prediction modelling using routine clinical parameters to stratify survival in malignant pleural mesothelioma patients undergoing cytoreductive surgery. Journal of Thoracic Oncology. 2019;**14**(2):288-293

[101] Gordon GJ, Dong L, Yeap BY, Richards WG, Glickman JN, Edenfield H, et al. Four-gene expression ratio test for survival in patients undergoing surgery for mesothelioma. Journal of the National Cancer Institute. 2009;**101**(9):678-686

[102] Gordon GJ, Rockwell GN, Godfrey PA, Jensen RV, Glickman JN, Yeap BY, et al. Validation of genomics-based prognostic tests in malignant pleural mesothelioma. Clinical Cancer Research. 2005;**11**(12):4406-4414

[103] Yeap BY, De Rienzo A, Gill RR, Oster ME, Dao MN, Dao NT, et al. Mesothelioma risk score: A new prognostic pretreatment, clinical-molecular algorithm for malignant pleural mesothelioma. Journal of Thoracic Oncology. 2021;**16**(11):1925-1935

[104] Billé A, Krug LM, Woo KM, Rusch VW, Zauderer MG. Contemporary analysis of prognostic factors in patients with unresectable malignant pleural mesothelioma. Journal of Thoracic Oncology. 2016;**11**(2):249-255

Chapter 5

Talc and Malignant Mesothelioma

Richard Kradin

Abstract

Malignant mesothelioma is a rare malignancy of serosal-lined tissues. It has been recognized since the last century that the majority of pleural mesotheliomas are caused by exposures to asbestos, a fibrous silicate mineral that was used extensively in the construction trades for its insulating properties. A previously unrecognized source of asbestos exposure is cosmetic talc that has been widely used for personal hygiene and other purposes by adults and children. Since 2014, more than 200 cases of mesothelioma have been reported in individuals, whose only known source of asbestos exposure was cosmetic talc. In this chapter the association of talc with malignant mesothelioma will be reviewed.

Keywords: mesothelioma, cosmetic talc, pleura, asbestos, tremolite, anthophyllite

1. Introduction

Malignant mesothelioma is a rare malignancy of serosal-lined tissues, including the pleura, peritoneum, tunica vaginalis, and pericardium. The disease was virtually unknown prior to the introduction of asbestos into the workplace and misattributed to metastatic carcinoma. Asbestos is a generic term that has been applied to six naturally occurring fibrous magnesium silicates that were used primarily for their insulating properties in the construction and other trades (**Table 1**). In 1960, when Wagner described 33 cases in workers and those living in proximity to crocidolite (blue asbestos) mine in South Africa [1]. Subsequent studies demonstrated that all commercially available forms of asbestos were capable of causing malignant mesothelioma (MM), with amphibole (needle-like) forms of asbestos being more carcinogenic on a per

Class	Type	Chemical formula
Serpentine	Chrysotile	$Mg_3(Si_2O_5)(OH)_4$
Amphibole	Amosite	$Fe_7Si_8O_{22}(OH)_2$
	Crocidolite	$Na_2Fe^{II}_3Fe^{III}_2Si_8O_{22}(OH)_2$
	Tremolite	$Ca_2Mg_5Si_8O_{22}(OH)_2$
	Actinolite	$Ca_2(Mg,Fe^{II})_5(Si_8O_{22})(OH)_2$
	Anthophyllite	$(Mg,Fe^{II})_7Si_8O_{22}(OH)_2$

Table 1.
Regulated asbestos by class, type, and chemical formula.

IntechOpen

fiber basis than chrysotile (serpentine). Due to the strength of association of asbestos and MM in epidemiological studies, the diagnosis of MM should "trigger" inquiry as to whether an individual may have been exposed to asbestos.

The prospective risk of developing mesothelioma is directly proportional to the dose (frequency/intensity/duration) of exposure. However, this refers to the *a priori* risk of developing disease and a low risk should not dissuade one from attributing a mesothelioma to asbestos when there is a history of past exposure. Approximately 10% of heavily exposed insulators have developed mesothelioma so that even heavy exposures do not necessarily lead to the development of disease [2]. At least four epidemiological studies have demonstrated that the risk of developing MM more than doubles following exposures as low as <0.1 f/cc-yr, and cases have been described following brief exposures [3]. Currently, no recognized safe level of occupational or paraoccupational exposure above background (~0.0001 f/cc) has been established. Due to the increased risk of developing MM following low-level exposures, asbestos has been banned by the European Union. However, its use in some products in the U.S. continues to be regulated with a current permissible exposure limit (PEL) of 0.1 f/cc over an 8 h time weighted average. Despite strict controls, regulatory agencies have predicted that even at this level there will be an excess, albeit small, risk of developing MM.

1.1 Clinical features, diagnostics, and treatment

The clinical features of pleural MM are largely stereotypic. Patients complain of cough, shortness of breath, chest pain, and weight loss as common presenting symptoms. Chest imaging generally shows a pleural effusion and nodular pleural thickening that extends circumferentially around the underlying lung. The diagnosis can be established by cytological evidence of malignancy in the pleural fluid or more commonly by pleural biopsy. The spectrum of pathologies include epithelioid and sarcomatoid variants, and the latter has a somewhat more aggressive clinical course. The diagnosis is generally confirmed by immunohistological staining. Positive tumor cell immunostaining for pancytokeratins, calretinin, WT-1, podoplanin (D2–40), CK7, CK5/6, is seen in the majority of cases with epithelioid features, whereas areas of sarcomatoid growth may lack expression of most mesothelial-associated antigens. The majority of epithelioid mesotheliomas also show loss of nuclear expression of BAP-1 and loss of *CDKN2A* [4].

The disease is virtually always lethal. Complete surgical extirpation is near impossible to achieve due to early invasion of chest wall and mediastinal structures. Current therapeutic interventions include pleurectomy/decortication with combination chemotherapy and/or immunotherapy. Life expectancy is less than two years with or without treatment in most studies [5].

1.2 Pathogenesis

With respect to causation, as individuals are often exposed repeatedly to asbestos, and to multiple sources of asbestos, the specific exposures responsible for the molecular events leading to MM cannot be ascertained. Rather, the cumulative exposure is considered to be the primary determinant of risk for developing MM. Even small amounts of an asbestos-containing material when disrupted can release millions of respirable microscopic asbestos fibers and a gram of asbestos includes more than a trillion fibers. Asbestos fibers are best visualized with transmission electron microscopy and cannot be reliably seen with standard light microscopy. Scanning electron microscopy underestimates asbestos fiber deposition. Fibers that are respirable and deposited in the lung can be transported via lymphatics to other serosal sites where they may cause disease [6, 7]. Fiber-burden analyses, an experimental technique used in an effort to assess asbestos fiber burden and type of fibers deposited is usually based on deposition within the lung, whereas the site of interest is the pleura which is rarely examined. Fiber-burden studies that focus on lung content also underestimate chrysotile content, as this fiber type has a short half-life (days to weeks) in the lung, whereas short fibers of chrysotile appear to persist in the pleura. Some asbestos fibers in the peripheral lung may penetrate the pleura and produce mutations in the lining mesothelial cells directly.

The pathways leading to asbestos-related malignancy are multifactorial. The vast majority of fibers (>90%) are cleared by the host defense mechanism that include nasal hairs, cough, swallowing, muco-ciliary clearance, and phagocytic cells. Nevertheless, those fibers that escape host defenses are capable of causing disease. Pathways leading to injury include direct injury to chromosomal DNA by asbestos fibers and the generation of free-radicals capable of producing genetic injury by inflammatory cells in response to fiber deposition in the pleura.

Much has been learned in recent years concerning the molecular genetics of MM carcinogenesis. Certain genes are frequently somatically mutated in the tumor cells of MM. These include *BAP-1, NF2, CDKN2A, p53*, mismatch repair genes, and others. In addition, there are families predisposed to developing MM, most notably those with heterozygous germline mutations in *BAP-1* [8]. However, biallelic mutations of *BAP-1* are seen in MM so that a second non-germline mutation must take place in the path towards malignant transformation [9]. Currently it appears that gene-environmental interactions are required for the development of MM and there is no compelling evidence that germline mutations are sufficient to cause MM in the absence of an environmental mutagen, most often asbestos.

2. Talc

Talc is a naturally occurring mineral mined from the earth. It is a hydrous magnesium silicate with chemical formula Mg3Si4O10(OH)2. Talc dominantly forms from the metamorphism of magnesian minerals such as serpentine, pyroxene, amphibole, and olivine, in the presence of carbon dioxide and water. This is known as "talc carbonation" and produces a suite of rocks known as talc carbonates.

Talc has been used extensively in industrial and pharmaceutical settings as well as in cosmetic powders. Whereas industrial talc varies in composition and may include a mixture of various mineral particles, cosmetic talc consists of platyform particles with only minor impurities (**Table 2**). Cosmetic talc has been mined throughout the world, with mines located in Italy, Vermont, North Carolina, Montana, Alabama, Korea, and China. Analyses of cosmetic talc from these sources have shown heterogeneous impurities including asbestiform tremolite, anthophyllite, actinolite, and chrysotile. The level of asbestos impurity varies but is usually less than 1% [10].

It is noteworthy that talc is the only commercial product that potentially includes both tremolite and/or anthophyllite and/or actinolite. Actinolite is not found in any commercial product other than talc. Tran et all have suggested that finding talc together with tremolite/actinolite/anthophyllite in fiber burden analyses of tissues is *prima facie* evidence of cosmetic talc use [11].

Mineral group	Name
Carbonate	Dolomite
	Magnesite
	Calcite
	Siderite
Phylosillicate	Chlorite
	Lizardite
	Mica
	Sepiolite
Amphibole	Tremolite
	Actinolite
	Anthophyllite
Tectosilicates	Quartz
	Feldspar
	Magnetite
	Rutile
	Manganese oxide
Sulfides	Pyrite
	Pentlandite
Other	Graphite

Table 2.
Minerals associated with talc.

The detection of asbestos within samples of cosmetic talc has been controversial and hindered by its presence as a low-level impurity. Identification depends on identifying asbestos fibers (aspect ratio > 3:1) and distinguishing them reliably from talc cleavage fragments. Although the earliest reports showing asbestos in talc were based on X-ray diffraction, accurate identification is optimally carried out by analytical transmission electron microscopy with either electron dispersive spectrometry or selected-area electron diffraction. Blount examined the amphibole content of high-grade cosmetic talc products from deposits in Vermont, Montana, North Carolina and Alabama using a centrifuge/optical method that enriches for amphibole fibers and found a uniformly low amphibole count that included both cleavage fragments and asbestiform fibers with aspect ratios >3:1 [12]. Other investigators have confirmed Blount's findings using the centrifuge/optical technique, [13] and a recent Federal Drug Administration analysis revealed chrysotile within a popular cosmetic talc product [14].

3. Mesothelioma and talc

Although asbestos was used primarily as an insulating material, it has been identified in other commercial products as well. In 1974, Rohl and Langer showed that

10 of 20 talc products, including baby powders, facial talcums, and pharmaceuticals, contained both tremolite and anthophyllite asbestiform structures [15]. This finding was contested by manufacturers, and went largely unnoticed by the medical community. However, in 2015 Gordon *et al* identified amphibole asbestos in a cosmetic talcum powder as well as in the lung tissue of a woman with MM who had no other known source of asbestos exposure [16]. The asbestos fibers were confirmed as anthophyllite and tremolite by electron dispersive spectrometry and by selected-area electron diffraction.

In 2019 Moline *et al* reported 33 cases of MM of the pleura and peritoneum associated with cosmetic talc exposure in subjects referred for medical-legal consultation [17]. In 2020, Emory, Maddox, and Kradin reported 75 additional subjects with MM who had been exposed to cosmetic talc [18]. In 2023, Moline, Patel, and Frank reported 166 additional cases of malignant mesothelioma diagnosed in cosmetic talc users [19]. 44 of these had potential or documented sources of asbestos exposure other than talc. 52/166 of the cases had diffuse peritoneal mesothelioma (DPM), with a similar percentage seen in men and women.

At the present time almost 300 cases of MM have been reported in the medical literature associated at least in part to cosmetic talc usage. Other than a somewhat younger age at time of diagnosis and an increased percentage of women, the clinical features and histology of these tumors has been indistinguishable from mesotheliomas produced by asbestos from other sources. However, due to the widespread availability and application of cosmetic talc in the community, it is possible that an unknown percentage of MM particularly in women previously labeled as "idiopathic" may have been attributable to cosmetic talc use [17].

Until the recent spate of cases of MM, it was thought that cosmetic talc, when used as intended, did not present a health hazard. But this position may not be justified based on the newly recognized cases of MM in talc users, although as will be discussed, it is likely that the prospective risk of developing MM from cosmetic talc use is low. The International Agency for Research on Cancer (IARC) states that asbestos contaminated talc is carcinogenic and should be treated as a potential carcinogen [20].

The argument that cosmetic talc is safe has been based on failure to identify cases of MM in cosmetic talc miners. A recent meta-analysis of six articles that included 5394 miners examined the incidence of MM and showed no increase, although there was a small increase in lung cancer and pneumoconiosis mortality [21]. Clinical trials to examine the risk of developing MM from the use of cosmetic talc have not been conducted and they may not be feasible for the following reasons. It is recognized that ~3000 new cases of mesothelioma occur in the U.S. each year. Although there are currently no data as to how many cases of MM are potentially attributable to cosmetic talc, a liberal "guesstimate" might be 10%, i.e., 300 cases/year. Estimating conservatively that perhaps half of the U.S. population (~150,000,000 individuals) has *ever* been exposed to cosmetic talc (CT), and assuming 300 new cases of MM potentially attributable to talc per year, one calculates that 0.0002% of the population would be expected to have a CT-associated MM. To detect a *single* case of malignant mesothelioma, ~500,000 subjects would need to be examined and that number would increase if the true incidence of CT-associated MM is less than 300.

Admittedly, the above calculation is crude, but its order of magnitude is likely approximately correct. While it does not account for the likely higher exposure levels to asbestos in cosmetic talc miners, it does suggest that screening an extremely large number of subjects would be necessary to detect cases of MM and to assess prospective

Bradford Hill criteria for assessing causality
1. Strength of association
2. Consistency of association
3. Specificity
4. Temporality
5. Biological gradient
6. Plausibility
7. Coherence
8. Experimental findings
9. Analogy
Hill argued that these were as important as finding statistical significance in an epidemiological study.

Table 3.
Criteria suggested by Sir Austin Bradford Hill that should be met in assessing causation.

risk. While one can conclude from this estimate that the incidence of MM due to cosmetic talc use is likely low, in a large population, cases can be expected to occur.

Kanarek and Liegel have argued that exposure to cosmetic talc containing asbestos meets the Bradford Hill criteria for causality of MM [22] (**Table 3**). As the ability of asbestos to cause MM is well established, epidemiological studies are not required to confirm this. Instead, the only justifiable role for an epidemiological study of cosmetic talc would be to establish the prospective risk to those exposed, not causation.

4. Cosmetic talc use

Cosmetic talc is a component of body powders, facial and eye makeups, and some animal flea powders [23]. Although asbestos is a trace impurity of cosmetic talc, concentrations of amphibole asbestos during the application of cosmetic talc powders have been measured at ~2.7–4.5 f/cc, which is orders of magnitude greater than current urban background levels (0.0001 f/cc) [13, 16]. It has been used primarily for personal hygiene after bathing but also in the diapering process of infants, as a dry deodorant, and as a dry shampoo. Some subjects report adding it to their shoes to reduce odor. Cosmetic talc is routinely used by barbers in hair salons where it is dusted on the neck area to prevent irritation. Twelve barbers were amongst the reported cases of MM, although a recent meta-analysis of 12 studies of barbers, hair stylists and cosmetologists suggests that their risk of developing disease may be low [24]. Unusual uses of cosmetic talc are occasionally reported. One subject with MM, as a young boy simulated an "ice skating" rink by pouring cosmetic talc over his living room floor. Under conditions like this, exposures to asbestos within talc may be considerable and result in increased risk for developing diseases, including MM, pleural plaques, and talcosis.

5. Demographics

The cases of talc associated MM have included both men and women with female predominance (~70%). The average age for both men and women has been in the early 60s [17–19]. The majority of MM have been pleural (~60%), but a higher-than-expected percentage have been women with peritoneal mesothelioma (~35%). The underlying genetics of these cases was not consistently available, although a small number of talc-associated MM have shown germline mutations in the *BAP-1* gene (unpublished data).

The published cases of talc-associated MM have all been identified through litigation. This may be attributable to the heightened consciousness related to the topic within the legal setting. While an uncertain percentage of all cases of MM are referred for litigation, it is likely high due to the level of publicity that surrounds the topic. In addition, physicians caring for patients with asbestos-related diseases may feel obliged to point out their option of pursuing compensation.

6. Conclusion

The recognition that cosmetic talc may be contaminated with asbestos has raised concerns in the medical community, regulatory agencies, and amongst consumers. Despite sporadic reports dating back to the 1970s, it has only been in the last decade that the potential for cosmetic talc to cause malignancies, including MM and ovarian cancer has been recognized.

Prior to this observation roughly 20% of MM in men and roughly half of MM in women were judged to be "idiopathic," i.e., it was not possible to identify a source of asbestos exposure. It is noteworthy that cases of talc-associated MM in the past would have been judged "idiopathic."

The identification of asbestos in cosmetic talc has had substantial economic impact and has triggered contentious ongoing litigation. Although the risk of developing cancer from cosmetic talc is apparently low, as MM is an incurable malignancy, this finding may justify seeking alternatives to its continued use. Increased awareness will require regulatory agencies to reexamine whether cosmetic talc products need to be regulated, labeled as potentially toxic, or banned for consumer usage.

Conflict of interest

The author has served as a compensated expert witness in talc litigation.

Author details

Richard Kradin
Massachusetts General Hospital, Harvard Medical School, Boston, MA, USA

*Address all correspondence to: richardkradin@gmail.com

References

[1] Wagner JC. Mesothelioma and mineral fibers. Cancer. 1986;**57**(10):1905-1911

[2] Selikoff IJ, Seidman H. Asbestos-associated deaths among insulation workers in the United States and Canada, 1967-1987. Annals of the New York Academy of Sciences. 1991;**643**:1-14

[3] Lacourt A et al. Occupational and non-occupational attributable risk of asbestos exposure for malignant pleural mesothelioma. Thorax. 2014;**69**(6):532-539

[4] Kradin RL. Understanding Pulmonary Pathology. New York: Academic Press; 2017

[5] Janes S, Alrifai D, Fennell D. Perspectives on the treatment of malignant pleural mesothelioma. New England Journal of Medicine. 2021;**385**:1207-1218

[6] Suzuki Y, Yuen SR. Asbestos tissue burden study on human malignant mesothelioma. Industrial Health. 2001;**39**(2):150-160

[7] Dodson RF, Atkinson MA. Measurements of asbestos burden in tissues. Annals of the New York Academy of Sciences. 2006;**1076**:281-291

[8] Carbone M et al. Mesothelioma: Scientific clues for prevention, diagnosis, and therapy. CA: A Cancer Journal for Clinicians. 2019;**69**(5):402-429

[9] Cheung M, Testa JR. BAP1, a tumor suppressor gene driving malignant mesothelioma. Translational Lung Cancer Research. 2017;**6**(3):270-278

[10] King H. Talc: The softest mineral. 2023. Available from: https://geology.com/minerals/talc.shtml

[11] Tran T et al. A critique of Helsinki criteria for using lung fiber levels to determine causation in mesothelioma cases. Annals of Global Health. 2021;**87**:1-13

[12] Blount A. Amphibole content of cosmetic and pharmaceutical talcs. Environmental Health Perspectives. 1991;**94**:225-230

[13] Steffen JE et al. Serous ovarian cancer caused by exposure to Asbestos and fibrous talc in cosmetic talc powders: A case series. Journal of Occupational and Environmental Medicine. 2020;**62**(2):e65-e77

[14] U.S. Food and Drug Administration. 18 Oct 2019. Available from: https://www.fda.gov/cosmetics/cosmetics-recalls-alerts/fda-advises-consumers-stop-using-certain-cosmetic-products

[15] Rohl AN, Langer AM. Identification and quantitation of asbestos in talc. Environmental Health Perspectives. 1974;**9**:95-109

[16] Gordon R, Fitzgerald S, Millette J. Asbestos in commercial cosmetic talcum powder as a cause of mesothelioma in women. International Journal of Occupational and Environmental Health. 2015;**21**(4):347-348

[17] Moline J et al. Mesothelioma associated with the use of cosmetic talc. Journal of Occupational and Environmental Medicine. 2020;**62**(1):11-17

[18] Emory TS, Maddox JC, Kradin RL. Malignant mesothelioma following repeated exposures to cosmetic talc: A case series of 75 patients. American Journal of Industrial Medicine. 2020;**63**(6):484-489

[19] Moline J, Patel K, Frank AL. Exposure to cosmetic talc and mesothelioma. Journal of Occupational Medical Toxicology. 2023;**18**(1):1

[20] IARC. Talc containing asbestiform fibers. 1987. Available from: https://publications.iarc.fr/Book-And-Report-Series/Iarc-Monographs-Supplements/Overall-Evaluations-Of-Carcinogenicity-An-Updating-Of-IARC-Monographs-Volumes-1-42-1987

[21] Ciocan C et al. Risk of mortality from respiratory malignant and non-malignant diseases among talc miners and millers: A systematic review and meta-analysis. Toxics. 2022;**10**(10)

[22] Kanarek MS, Liegel JC. Asbestos in talc and mesothelioma: Review of the causality using epidemiology. Medical Research Archives. May 2020;**8**(5). DOI: 10.18103/mra.v8i5.2097. ISSN 2375-1924. Available from: https://esmed.org/MRA/mra/article/view/2097

[23] Tran T et al. A critique of Helsinki criteria for using lung Fiber levels to determine causation in mesothelioma cases. Annals of Global Health. 2021;**87**(1):73

[24] Lewis RC et al. Occupational exposure to cosmetic talc and mesothelioma in barbers, hairdressers, and cosmetologists: A systematic review of the epidemiology. Toxicology and Industrial Health. 2023:**39**(10):564-582. DOI: 10.1177/07482337231191162

Section 4

Cutting Edge in Pleural Pathology: New Entities

Chapter 6

Pleuroparenchymal Fibroelastosis and Serositis as Pleural Complications after Hematopoietic Stem Cell and Lung Transplantation

Pat Arndt

Abstract

Pulmonary complications after hematopoietic stem cell transplantation (HSCT) and lung transplantation involve both infectious and non-infectious etiologies. Although infectious complications are much more common, with literature describing their clinical presentation, diagnosis, treatments, and outcome, the non-infectious complications are less well understood. The overall incidence of non-infectious complications after transplantation is much less frequent, and in some instances is rare. Another challenge with the non-infectious complications is that there are no key biomarkers for establishing a diagnosis, with the need to rely on clinical symptoms and radiologic findings. Treatments are generally non-existent or are empiric in nature. Another important feature of the non-infectious complications is that they are generally chronic in duration and are associated with high rates of mortality as well as morbidity, with a significant effect on patients' quality of life. An understanding of the pleural associated pulmonary complications after HSCT and lung transplantation is necessary for pulmonologists, transplant physicians, and Internal/Family medicine providers. Improvement in the knowledge of underlying mechanisms for pleural based pulmonary complications after HSCT and lung transplantation are drastically needed design of targeted therapies for treatment. In this review, we will discuss the post-transplant pleural based complications of serositis and pleuroparenchymal fibroelastosis.

Keywords: serositis, pleuroparenchymal fibroelastosis, transplant, complications, hematopoietic stem cell transplant, lung

1. Introduction

Hematopoietic stem cell transplantation (HSCT) is commonly performed to treat hematological malignancies and has also been used to treat a select group of, non-hematologic malignancies and genetic disorders [1, 2]. Recent data shows that more than 150,000 HSCT are performed each year worldwide [1, 2]. Similarly, the number of lung transplantations for end stage lung disease is increasing yearly [3, 4]. With the continued relaxation of the age restriction for eligibility for lung transplantation and use of pre-transplant respiratory support with extracorporeal membrane oxygenation (ECMO) as a bridge to successful transplant, the number of transplantations per year is likely to increase [4]. Accordingly, as the overall number of patients undergoing hematopoietic or lung transplantation increases, the number of patients who need to be cared for long-term after transplant is increasing. As many of these patients resume their normal lives after transplant, residing in geographic areas distal to the transplant centers and tertiary care medical centers, primary care providers and sub-specialists not accustomed to caring for post-HSCT and lung transplant patients will need to oversee their routine post-transplant care as well as be the initial providers to assess and treat these patients when they present with complications after transplant. An understanding of the post-HSCT and lung transplant complications that occur in these patients is vital to these providers. Although HSCT and lung transplants are lifesaving, the post-transplant course for patients can be challenging due to both infectious and non-infectious complications, with the lungs being a frequent target. Specifically for HSCT, the lung is the most common organ involved in post-transplant complications where 30–60% of patients undergoing HSCT develop lung complications [1, 5, 6]. Similar findings are also observed after lung transplant wherein many of the acute complications are related to post-operative challenges including bleeding, acute respiratory failure, and allograft ischemia/reperfusion [7–9]. In both of these patient populations, pulmonary infectious complications are most common in the early phases after transplantation due to the high levels of immunosuppression needed to prevent rejection, however pulmonary infections can occur at any time after HSCT or lung transplantation while the patient remains on immunosuppressive medications [10–15]. In addition to infectious complications, complications involving the pleura also occur after HSCT and lung transplantation with presentations of pleural effusions, pneumothorax, and hemothorax [7, 8, 16–22]. The reported incidence of pleural complications after lung transplantation is 22–45% whereas those after HSCT are much less [7, 8, 16, 23]. Whilst many of these pleural complications are related to other clinical conditions (infection, cardiac dysfunction, acute renal disease, volume overload, or trauma) with treatment directed at these conditions, other less common, poorly understood, and difficult to treat pleural complications can occur after HSCT and lung transplantation. This review will discuss two of these rare pleural based post HSCT and lung transplant complications, serositis and pleuroparenchymal fibroelastosis (PPFE). Serositis and PPFE are pleural based complications typically seen much later after HSCT or lung transplant with variable time frame of onset and disease progression [7, 8, 18–21]. At present, neither of these non-infectious post-transplant complications have effective treatments with the typical disease process progressing over time leading to chronic respiratory symptoms, additional complications, an overall decreased quality of life, and diminished life expectancy. In this review we will focus on these two pleural associated complications after HSCT and lung transplant and will describe their clinical presentation, objective clinical and radiographic findings, what is known of their underlying pathophysiology and potential underlying etiologies, establishment of a diagnosis, and current therapies directed at these complications. We will also discuss the current research being done for each condition to increase the understanding of risk factors, pathophysiologic mechanisms for disease, disease associations, potential biomarkers, and ongoing efforts to identify novel avenues for therapy.

2. Serositis

Serositis is as recently described but poorly understood late pulmonary complication seen after HSCT and lung transplantation. Pleural and pericardial effusions are frequently seen shortly after lung and hematopoetic stem cell transplantation but are generally gone within a few months after transplant ([16, 18, 19] and unpublished observations). For post-HSCT patients the underlying cause for these effusions are poorly understood, with infection seldom an identified etiology, and are likely related to volume overload due to the need for transfusion support during the pre-engraftment time period. For post-lung transplant patients, early pleural effusions are associated with the surgical procedure and include hemothorax, post-surgical cardiac dysfunction or volume overload, increased alveolar capillary permeability, or transient disruption of lymphatic drainage directly secondary to the lung transplant procedure but less likely infection [7, 9, 16, 17]. Pleural effusions in post lung transplant patients typically resolve within the first few weeks after transplant with a median time of 19.4 days (range 5–52 days) as seen in the study by Ferrer et al. [16], and do not recur unless initially due to bleeding, infection, or other pleural complication due to the lung transplant surgery procedure [16]. Effusions seen after this time period are much less common in these patients [16, 17]. Similar to the effusions seen earlier in the post-transplant course, these effusions can be similarly caused by infection, cardiac dysfunction, or volume overload. Finally, late pleural or pericardial effusions in the late post-transplant time period after HSCT or lung transplant may be related to malignancy, including post-transplant lymphoproliferative disease (PTLD), [7, 9, 18, 19, 24]. All of these potential causes of late onset pleural effusions need to be carefully evaluated and excluded [7, 8, 18, 19, 24]. For post-HSCT patients, however, effusions with a negative work-up for other causes from day 100 onward after HSCT are thought to be part of chronic GvHD (cGvHD) and are termed serositis [18–21]. Although no definitive term for serositis is currently used after lung transplantation, in one study 41.5% of the late pleural effusions after lung transplantation were termed idiopathic after undergoing routine diagnostic analysis and can be therefore also grouped into likely serositis [9]. By definition, serositis is described as inflammation of the serosal surfaces in the peritoneum, pleural, and pericardial cavities [18, 19, 21, 25, 26]. It has been previously associated with numerous systemic disorders and drug or chemical exposures [25–28]. Additionally, it has been described prominently in autoimmune conditions such as rheumatoid arthritis, systemic lupus erythematosus (SLE), and inflammatory bowel disease (IBD) [25–29]. Serositis after HSCT is a rare complication occurring in <5% of all patients after allogeneic HSCT, however the true incidence is not known as only a few larger studies are available outlining this condition [18, 19]. At our institution, the overall incidence of post-HSCT serositis in the patients we follow is around 4% (Unpublished observations) which is similar to the findings by Leonard et al. that reported 23 cases of serositis in 894 HSCT recipients over a 16 year period giving an incidence of less than 3% [19] and by Modi et al. confirming these observations by reporting an incidence of less than 2% [18]. Taken together these studies suggest a prevalence of 2–4% after HSCT. Regarding potential demographic associations for post-HSCT serositis, in contrast to SLE associated serositis, where male sex was an independent risk factor for pleural effusion [28], a strong age or gender predilection for cGvHD-associated serositis has not been described in the literature or in our clinical experience, wherein neither age, gender, nor type of underlying malignancy were found to be possible risk factors for the development of post-HSCT cGvHD-associated serositis ([18, 19] and Unpublished observation). For post-HSCT serositis most cases occur in the setting of established pre-existing cGvHD, although rarely serositis can be the initial presentation of cGvHD and can be seen in those that underwent autologous transplantation who do not experience cGvHD ([18, 19], and unpublished observations). As stated above, unlike other non-infectious pulmonary complications after HSCT, serositis is a late pulmonary complication after HSCT and is associated with cGvHD. A significant lag time occurs between the initial onset of cGvHD and the diagnosis of pleural or pericardial effusions associated serositis [18, 19, 22]. Furthermore, in most cases, retrospective review of imaging shows the onset of small pleural or pericardial effusions in post-HSCT patients with cGvHD that remain asymptomatic much earlier in the course with the development of symptomatic disease only occurring later (up to over 200 days) (18 and Unpublished observations). These small pleural effusions in post-HSCT patients with cGvHD are usually identified by radiologic imaging (chest x-ray or CT scan) done for other clinical reasons. In our experience, 25% of our patients had pleural effusions that remained completely asymptomatic during follow-up prior to a confirmed diagnosis of cGvHD serositis. In contrast, 33% of our patients had effusions that remained clinically insignificant for up to 241 days after their occurrence until presenting with symptoms related to the effusions and the diagnosis of serositis. As such, the identification of small asymptomatic pleural or pericardial effusions by imaging in post-HSCT patients requires close clinical follow-up for the development of respiratory symptoms with instructions to patients to report respiratory symptoms of shortness of breath or cough. To our knowledge no prospective study has been done to follow post-HSCT patients with cGvHD for the occurrence of pleural or pericardial effusions to identify risk factors, biomarkers, or treatment interventions earlier in the disease course.

As stated above, no definitive description or diagnosis for post lung transplant associated serositis exists but review of the literature of pleural or pericardial effusions after lung transplant describes the occurrence of non-classifiable effusions later in the post lung transplant course that would be consistent with a diagnosis of serositis [8, 9]. In these situations, infection, hemothorax, and malignancy have all been excluded using traditional clinical methods. In the large retrospective study by Tang et al., 26% of their patients developed pleural effusions with most of these patients developing pleural effusions in the early post-transplant course, reported as up to 9 months [8]. The exact number who developed late pleural effusions (after 9 months) following transplantation was not provided in that study [8]. In that study, there was no association of the development of a pleural effusion with acute rejection [8]. However, having a pleural effusion was associated with a decrease in survival [8]. In the retrospective review by Joean et al., 9.2% of their patients required thoracentesis for a pleural effusion after lung transplant [9]. Their patients were nearly equally divided into early and late onset pleural effusions (41% occurring late) with a definition of late being more than 6 months after transplant. Furthermore, 24% of early and 17% of late effusions had an indeterminate etiology after biochemical and microbiologic analysis suggesting that they may be related to pleural inflammation associated with serositis [9]. Based on the above studies, after lung transplantation there appears to be a bimodal time distribution to the development of pleural effusions with many occurring 6 months after transplant [8, 9, 16]. The etiology of these pleural effusion are not completely understood but may be related to serositis [8, 9, 16].

2.1 Clinical presentation

The clinical presentation of patients with symptomatic serositis after HSCT or lung transplantation depends on the organ involved. Presentation can be with shortness of breath of an acute or sub-acute duration, chest discomfort, abdominal fullness, light headedness, or dizziness due to accumulating fluid in the pleural, pericardial, or peritoneal, spaces [9, 16, 18, 19]. With pleural effusions, patients may also present with cough, that is dry in character, as well as chest pressure or the inability to take a deep breath. Most concerning are patients presenting with the rapid accumulation of fluid in the pericardial space leading to tamponade or in the pleural space causing acute respiratory failure [30, 31]. These patients require immediate evacuation of the fluid for stabilization. However, typically for pleural effusions after HSCT, based, on our experience and the literature, effusions increase over several months before patients develop symptoms and infrequently require emergent drainage for symptom control ([18, 19], and unpublished observations).

2.2 Pathophysiology and potential biomarkers for post-HSCT and lung transplant serositis

The underlying pathophysiology of post-HSCT and lung transplant induced serositis is poorly understood. Due to the rarity of this complication, only limited investigations have been undertaken into the pathogenesis and mechanism of disease either at the time of onset or during progression. At present there are a limited number of clinical markers available to predict those at an increased risk for developing serositis or that are useful to assess the potential for progressive disease and a poor clinical outcome. In contrast to SLE associated serositis, where male sex was identified as an independent risk factor for pleural effusions [28], a strong age or gender predilection for cGvHD-associated serositis has not been described, either in the literature or in our clinical observations ([18, 19] and unpublished observations). This is also true for the type of underlying malignancy requiring HSCT. Our observations further support these findings as neither age, gender, nor type of underlying malignancy were found to be possible risk factors for the development of post-HSCT cGvHD-associated serositis (unpublished observations). However for HSCT, donor type may be important. Seber et al. [32] in their study of post-HSCT serositis reported that 66.6% of unexplained effusions occurred in mismatched and unrelated donors in association with both acute and chronic GvHD. In our group of post-HSCT patients with serositis four patients (33.3%) received transplants from unrelated donors, out of which three had very severe serositis, with one succumbing to the disease (unpublished observations). Our findings therefore support those seen by Seber et al. [32]. Taken together, having an unrelated donor may be a risk factor for the development of serositis after HSCT. In addition, although studies have not described an association between the conditioning regimen and post-HSCT serositis, an increased incidence of acute and chronic GvHD [33] and constrictive pericarditis [34] has been reported in patients receiving TBI as a part of their conditioning regimen. All but one of the patients that we have seen who developed cGvHD pleural effusions after HSCT received TBI (91.6%). Thus, TBI may also be a possible risk factor for the onset serositis in patients with severe cGvHD.

At present there are no serum or pleural/pericardial fluid biomarkers to assist in the diagnosis, risk stratification, or use to target therapy or predict outcomes in patients with serositis after HSCT or lung transplantation. Regarding post-HSCT associate serositis, one study suggested that an acute decrease in serum albumin or increase in circulating monocytes may allow for identification of patients at risk for serositis after HSCT but this has not been followed up upon (19 Leonard). In other reports viral respiratory infections have been suggested to trigger the onset of serositis after HSCT [18]. In our patients we have seen this association in a small number but these findings have not been consistent across our whole patient population (unpublished observations). In contrast, for lung transplant patients that develop late onset pleural effusions, no studies to our knowledge have been undertaken to explore possible biomarkers. Furthermore, no published reports have extensively characterized the pleural or pericardial fluid in post-HSCT with serositis or post lung transplant patients that develop late onset pleural effusions, apart from a description of routine biochemical testing to determine exudative or transudative effusions by Lights criteria and exclusion of infection. A more extensive analysis of pleural or pericardial fluid from serositis patients may point to potential mechanisms underlying the pathogenesis of this complication and allow for the design of targeted therapies and predictors of outcomes.

2.3 Treatment for post-transplant serositis

In regards to treatment for serositis after transplantation, no clinical trials have been published outlining management of serositis after HSCT or lung transplant. At present treatment is focused on the drainage of symptomatic effusions for alleviation of symptoms and determination of other causes. Specifically for post-HSCT serositis associated pleural effusions, augmentation in immunosuppression using corticosteroids, tacrolimus and/or sirolimus has been attempted to prevent fluid re-accumulation [18, 19]. Other modalities tried have included extracorporeal photophoresis, etanercept, and rituximab [18] with variable success. Although an increase in the immunosuppression regimen was successful in a majority of post-HSCT patients with serositis treated by Modi et al., this approach was only effective in a quarter of our patients ([18] and Unpublished observation). For those unresponsive to an increase in immunosuppression, treatment is generally repeated procedures for fluid drainage to obtain symptom control. As these effusions are typically chronic in duration, this approach is sub-optimal to control patients' symptoms and requires frequent invasive procedures. Pleurodesis, involving the chemical irritation of the pleural space leading to adhesion of the visceral and parietal pleura, has been shown to be effective in a few patients with post-transplant serositis that has been recurrent [35]. The large volume of fluid associated with these pleural effusions, and the rapid re-accumulation that is typically seen, limits the effectiveness of this treatment modality. As stated above, although serositis as a cause for recurrent or non-resolving pleural effusions has not been explicitly described in post lung transplant patients, up to 41% of late onset effusions have been determined to be non-specific and therefore potentially serositis [9]. Detailed management of these non-specific late onset pleural effusions after lung transplant have not been described in the literature. Further research is necessary to determine the risk factors and underlying mechanisms leading to serositis after HSCT and lung transplantation in order to design effective treatments and improve patient outcomes.

3. PPFE

3.1 Overview

In addition to serositis, another rare and poorly understood pleural complication after HSCT and lung transplant is pleuroparenchymal fibroelastosis (PPFE). In the most recent review of the idiopathic interstitial pneumonias by the American Thoracic Society in 2013, PPFE was classified as a separate entity [36]. The disease was initially described by Amitani as an upper lobe predominant pleural based disease distinct from apical cap disease and termed pulmonary upper lobe fibrosis (PULF) [37]. It was later renamed pleuroparenchymal fibroelastosis (PPFE) by Frankel in their case series of patients with that name now established to describe the disease [38]. Since its initial description, the number of cases of PPFE continues to increase [36–39]. At present the diagnosis of PPFE is determined by the distinct radiographic pattern seen on chest X-ray or CT imaging as there is no specific definitive biomarker or test to establish the diagnosis apart from the radiographic description [40, 41]. Establishing a diagnosis of PPFE in post HSCT or lung transplant patients is important to avoid unnecessary or harmful procedures, to assess for the development of complications, and to provide information to patients and family members regarding the typical clinical course and survival. Below we will discuss the incidence, risk factors, clinical presentation, diagnostic work-up, present state of biomarkers, treatment and outcomes for PPFE with a focus on that which occurs after HSCT or lung transplantation.

3.2 Incidence of PPFE

Pleuroparenchymal fibroelastosis after HSCT or lung transplant is an uncommon to rare complication with specific differences in prevalence between the two groups. The overall prevalence of PPFE after HSCT is 0.28–3.3% [42–44] with a much higher prevalence rate (7.54–15%) seen after lung transplant [42, 45]. The reason for these significant differences in prevalence between the two groups is unknown but may point to specific risk factors or infectious or non-infectious exposure causing PPFE in each group. These differences remain unknown. For both post HSCT and lung transplantation, the onset of PPFE is much later in the course after transplant. Specifically for HSCT, unlike the other long term non-infectious pulmonary complications which occur within 100 days to 2 years after transplant, PPFE occurs much later with a median time to diagnosis of 6.9 years, with a wide time range (0.25–17.9 years) [10, 11, 13, 15, 17, 22, 42, 44, 46, 47]. This wide range in time to onset brings up the question if the PPFE diagnosed at the extreme ends of the time spectrum are the same or are different disease processes. At present it is unclear if an earlier manifestation is a separate and distinct disease process or if the etiologic cause is different than those diagnosed much later with PPFE. No studies to date have identified differences in exposures or potential risk factors between the two groups. For PPFE after lung transplant, the reason for the higher prevalence is unknown. As PPFE after lung transplant is combined in those with the restrictive allograft syndrome (RAS) subtype of chronic lung allograft dysfunction (CLAD), it makes it challenging to isolate it as a specific disease process when reviewing studies to determine individual risk factors or true prevalence [48–50].

Specifically for post-HSCT PPFE, the disease is mostly confined to those who have undergone allogeneic transplant, although a few cases are seen in patients who received an autologous transplant [22, 42]. As such, PPFE may be another manifestation of chronic graft versus host disease (cGvHD) and thereby suggesting similar pathophysiology for disease onset. However, as most other organ involvement of cGvHD occurs shortly after 100 days post-transplant and PPFE occurs much later, the underlying cause for PPFE may be unique compared to cGvHD as a whole. Typically post-HSCT patients that develop PPFE have established lung associated cGvHD (i.e. bronchiolitis obliterans syndrome (BOS), based on several studies and the experience at our institution ([22, 43, 46, 47, 51], unpublished observations) with the co-existence of BOS in patients diagnosed with PPFE being high at 47–100% [22, 46, 47, 51]. Taken together these findings suggest a similar underlying etiology and pathophysiology for BOS and PPFE. However mention needs to be made that as the average time to onset for BOS and PPFE after HSCT are different (BOS 1.5 years vs. PPFE 6.9 years) there may still be unique differences in the underlying cause and pathophysiology between the two entities. This is also true for differences seen in the incidence of the two diseases where BOS occurs in 5–10% of post-HSCT patients, but PPFE only occurs in a much smaller group of 0.2–0.3% of all patients undergoing allogeneic HSCT [18, 19, 46, 47]. This suggest the possibility of a "two hit" pathophysiology.

Similar to after HSCT, a similar entity to PPFE has been described in patients who have undergone lung transplantation [45, 52, 53]. However, unlike in post-HSCT patients, PPFE or PPFE-like lesions are grouped into the sub-category of restrictive allograft syndrome (RAS) under the broader post-lung transplant complication of chronic lung allograft dysfunction (CLAD), which includes the classic post-lung transplant chronic rejection entity of bronchiolitis obliterans syndrome (BOS) as well as the newer entity of RAS [48–50]. This makes the specific investigation of PPFE more challenging in these specific patients. A PPFE like disease in post lung transplant patients was initially described from researchers from the Toronto and Duke lung transplant groups upon a retrospective review of their post lung transplant patients over a 10 year time frame [52, 53]. In their study, the onset of an upper lobe predominant fibrotic lung disease occurred in 1.9% of their patients with a range of onset of 0.41–8 years and a median time to onset of 1.9 years. Similar to as was described above for post HSCT, the range of onset for PPFE after lung transplant is quite wide. In post-lung transplant patients the progression of PPFE appears to be quicker than after HSCT where in one study the calculated upper lobe volume loss was 45% over time as assessed by CT imaging [52]. Development of a pneumothorax was also frequent in this patient group with 71% developing a pneumothorax during follow-up [52]. On pulmonary function testing lung volumes were decreased, as would be expected with a fibrotic lung disease. In addition, in most patients the disease progressed slowly with radiographic findings present for several months prior to the onset of clinical symptoms [52, 53]. Collectively these findings are similar to those in post-HSCT patients that develop PPFE. As mentioned above, since these initial descriptions of PPFE after lung transplant, PPFE or PPFE-like findings after lung transplant have been grouped into the restrictive allograft syndrome, a poorly understood post transplant complication that was officially listed as a complication diagnosis by the International Society of Heart and Lung transplantation (ISHLT) in their update in 2019 [48]. Restrictive allograft syndrome occurs in 30–35% of patients who undergo lung transplantation and is present alone as a form of chronic rejection or is seen co-existing with bronchiolitis obliterans syndrome (BOS) [48–50, 54].

PPFE is a subset within the group of RAS without clear distinctions of specific groups within RAS identified by ISHLT [48, 49, 54].

3.3 Etiology and risk factors for PPFE after HSCT or lung transplantation

The cause of PPFE after HSCT or lung transplant is currently unknown (**Table 1**). For post-HSCT PPFE two possibilities have specifically been discussed, adverse reaction to chemotherapy or radiation used to treat the underlying disease or during the conditioning regimen prior to undergoing HSCT. Chemotherapeutic agents that have been implicated in causing PPFE include cyclophosphamide, and carmustine, which are alkylating agents [39, 47, 51, 55]. Taking away from these agents as possible causes for PPFE is that the overall incidence of PPFE after HSCT is very low whereas the number of transplant patients receiving alkylating agents is very high. In addition the long duration between the time of receiving alkylating chemotherapy and the onset of PPFE, which averages several years, lessens the potential association. Whole body irradiation, used during the conditioning period prior to HSCT, has been examined as a possible etiology for the later development PPFE but as only a few such treated patients later develop PPFE it is an unlikely causative agent [39, 47]. Similar to use of chemotherapeutic agents, An additional cause for both post HSCT, as well as lung transplant recipients, in developing PPFE are respiratory infections, particularly viral infections that occur after transplant [39, 42, 48, 51, 53, 55]. This makes clinical sense and would explain how PPFE can occur at all times post-transplant but particularly later in the course. All types of infections have been suggested to lead to PPFE after HSCT including viral, bacterial, and atypical pathogens. Interestingly there have been recent descriptions of an association of infection with atypical Mycobacteria infection and the development of PPFE in both HSCT and lung transplant patients [53, 56, 57]. Interestingly, this association has been seen both in non-transplant patients with atypical Mycobacteria infection who go on to develop PPFE and those diagnosed with PPFE that also were found to be infected with atypical Mycobacteria [56, 57]. Two large retrospective studies in those with atypical Mycobacterial infection showed the prevalence of PPFE was 11.9–26.3% [56, 57]. To date, however, the association of atypical Mycobacteria infection and PPFE in post HSCT or lung transplant patients has not been extensively examined with only a few case reports or isolated patient reports describing a co-association. At present no infectious cause for PPFE in post-HSCT or lung transplant patients has been identified. A lack of an animal model for PPFE limits the future exploration of a potential link between pulmonary infection and the later development of PPFE. Published cases that have implicated infections as a cause for PPFE in those have undergone HSCT have not provided details of infection type, nor the timing and duration of the infection prior to the development of PPFE [39, 42]. As respiratory infections are common in all patients, and especially after HSCT due to

Etiologies of pleuroparenchymal fibroelastosis
Idiopathic
Chemotherapy (e.g. cyclophosphamide, carmustine)
Radiation therapy
Respiratory infection—viral, atypical mycobacterium
Alloreactive inflammatory response

Table 1.
Listed above are the current known etiologies for PPFE.

an immunocompromised state, this deflects that respiratory infections are a cause for PPFE after HSCT as PPFE is very rare. In addition, in the studies suggesting a connection between respiratory infections and PPFE, the timing from a purported respiratory infection and PPFE is long, sometimes measured in years, and there is a lack of details describing the severity of the respiratory infection or the duration of the illness [42, 51].

Similar to post-HSCT PPFE, the etiology for RAS, and in particular PPFE, after lung transplant have not been determined. Etiologic investigation after lung transplant has encompassed a broader examination for the cause of chronic lung rejection after lung transplant (aka CLAD). These have included allograft rejection, humoral immunity, gastroesophogeal reflux disease (GERD), and infections [48, 50]. In addition, on reviewing demographics, no clear risk factors have been identified when examining age, sex, reason for transplant, surgical or post-surgical hospital course or complications, or medications [49, 54]. To date, no specific studies have been undertaken in a group of patients with RAS with predominant features of PPFE to determine specific etiologic factors. For CLAD and RAS as a whole, possible etiologic factors examined have included post-transplant hospital course, pre- and post-transplant immunosuppressive medications, GERD with aspiration, airway irritant exposure, rejection, and infections [48, 50, 53, 58]. The development of acute respiratory failure with the presence of diffuse alveolar damage (DAD) on lung biopsy results greater than 3 months after transplant correlated with the onset of RAS [48, 58, 59]. Similar findings of DAD in patients who have developed RAS was also seen by Ofek et al. [49]. Importantly these findings of DAD were observed in RAS patients who specifically were found to have PPFE with these findings present one or more years prior to the diagnosis of RAS [52, 53]. Taken together, this suggests that acute inflammation, and its effects may be a risk factor for PPFE. In addition, several studies have shown that pro-inflammatory mediators are increased in RAS patients including cytokines (Interleukins 5, 6, 8, CXCL10, and 1β), alarmins, and neutrophil elastase [48, 59–67]. Further suggesting that acute inflammation and possibly the development of DAD may predispose to the development of PPFE. The potential role of these pro-inflammatory mediators will be discussed below further under Biomarkers. Interestingly, levels of vascular endothelial growth factor (VEGF) is decreased in RAS patients [48]. This finding correlates with the observation of vascular injury on lung biopsies from patients with RAS and PPFE [67] and the decrease in vascular perfusion on ventilation perfusion scans taken on patients with an upper lobe predominant fibrosis after lung transplant [53]. Taken together, this suggests that a vascular injury after lung transplantation may place a patient at a higher risk for the development of RAS and therefore PPFE. The specific role of VEFGF in the development of PPFE after lung transplant has not been specifically examined. In regards to an alloimmune response as the cause of RAS and PPFE after lung transplant several avenues have been investigated. There has been no correlation for the development of RAS/PPFE and the use of immunosuppressive medications after transplant [50]. In contrast, the possibility that the presence of donor associated antibodies and antibody mediated rejection (AMR) and the development of RAS/PPFE have been investigated by several groups. In the study by Todd et al., there was an increased incidence of newly detected DSA that correlated to the onset of RAS [68]. Similar findings were reported by Verleden et al. in their group of patients [69]. These findings potentially fit with the observation of an increase in total immunoglobulin G levels in post-lung transplant patients that developed RAS [48]. The presence of GERD was thought be strongly associated with CLAD, and in particular BOS, based on lung biopsies showing multinucleated giant cells and lipid laden macrophages suggestive of chronic aspiration and clinical improvement in those who underwent fundoplication [48, 50, 53]. However, this has been not thought to definitively be a cause of RAS/PPFE. Finally, post-transplant infectious complications, similar to post-HSCT, have been examined as a potential cause for RAS/PPFE in patients who have undergone lung transplantation but no clear association has emerged. As discussed above for PPFE after HSCT, infection with atypical Mycobacteria has been suggested to be as cause of RAS/PPFE after lung transplantation. In the series by Pakhale et al. 5 patients had cultures positive for atypical Mycobacteria, with only two having positive cultures prior to the presence of radiographic changes [53]. As these patients did not have clinical disease suggestive of an atypical Mycobacterial infection, this was not felt to be an active infection and was not treated and accordingly was not felt to be the definite cause of PPFE.

3.4 Clinical presentation

The clinical presentation of PPFE after HSCT or RAS/PPFE after lung transplant is similar to cases from other etiologies or those considered to be idiopathic (**Table 2**). Presentations are of progressive shortness of breath and cough [22, 43, 45, 47, 52,53]. In the majority of cases the cough is non-productive with the shortness of breath slowly progressive over time with the diagnosis of PPFE commonly made several years after the onset of symptoms, with the an average time of 2.5 years, although the time from symptom onset to diagnosis is broad (0.5–6 years) [43, 52–54, 70]. As such a low level of suspicion for PPFE or Restrictive allograft syndrome (RAS)/PPFE must be maintained to ensure close clinical follow-up for diagnosis. Earlier identification may allow for quicker intervention or prevention of disease progression. Patients frequently have chest pain that is pleuritic in nature but this is not seen in all patients with PPFE [22, 39, 70]. In contrast, extrathoracic symptoms are unusual

Diagnostic criteria for pleuroparenchymal fibroelastosis (PPFE)
Symptoms
Shortness of breath/dyspnea on exertion—progressive in nature
Chest pain
Cough—dry
Radiologic imaging
Upper lobe predominance
Pleural thickening
Subpleural fibrotic bands with radiation toward hilum
Lower lobe interstitial changes—variable occurrence and pattern
Pneumothorax
Lung physiology—pulmonary function testing
Decrease in forced vital capacity (FVC)
Increased residual volume (RV)/total lung capacity (TLC) ratio
Preserved diffusion capacity (DLCO)
Desaturation uncommon until later stages
Lung histology
Routine lung biopsy not recommended
Upper lobe fibrotic bands
Pleural thickening
Lower lobe usual interstitial pneumonitis (UIP) or non-specific interstitial pneumonitis (NSIP) pattern

Table 2.
Clinical, radiographic, and histologic patterns in establishing a diagnostic of PPFE.

in patients with post-HSCT PPFE or RAS/PPFE after lung transplant. Patients typically have a history of weight loss with a low body mass index (BMI) with the low BMI used as one diagnostic criteria for PPFE and which can help in differentiating PPFE from the other types of IIP [43, 45, 70]. With an upper lobe predominance for PPFE causing fibrosis in the upper lobes with resultant hilar retraction, patients with PPFE develop a flattened chest or platythorax (**Figure 1**) [43, 45, 70]. Platythorax severity is calculated via the longitudinal versus transverse ratio at the level of the 6th

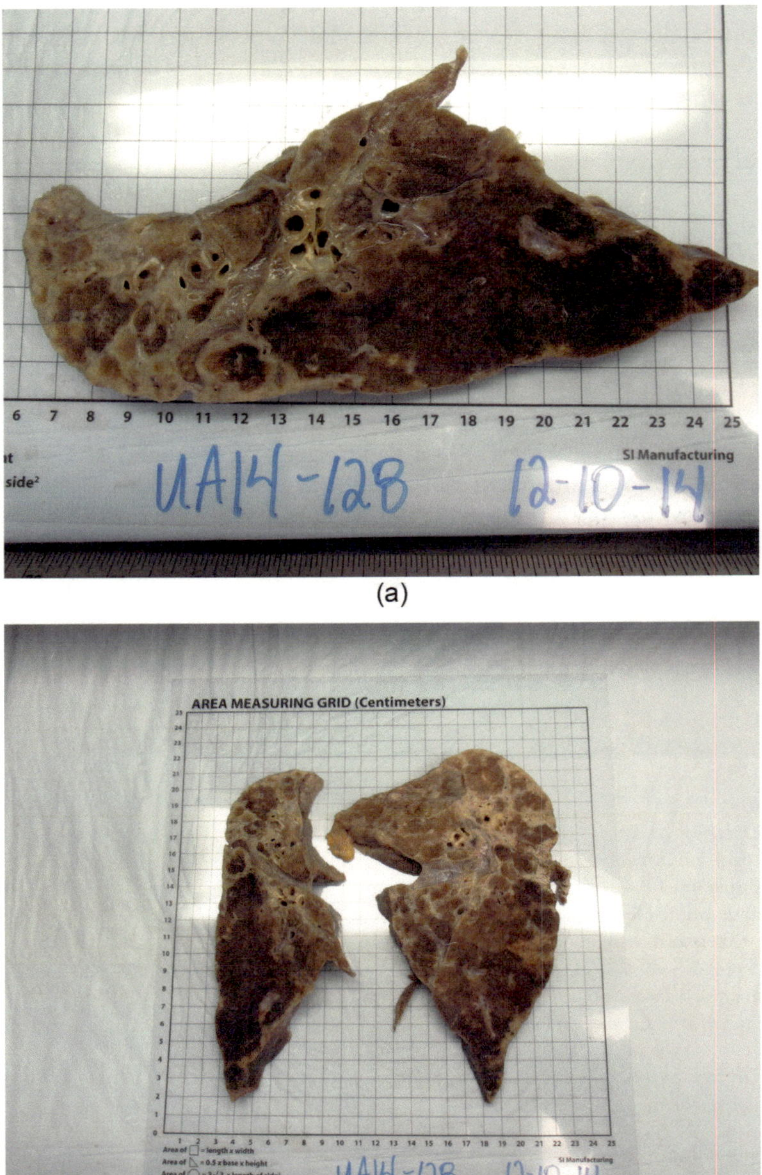

(a)

(b)

Figure 1.
Lungs obtained at autopsy from a patient with PPFE. Note fibrotic bands leading to hilum and upper lobe predominance of these bands.

thoracic vertebra [43]. On lung examination, the presence of crackles are less common in patients with PPFE, compared to those with idiopathic pulmonary fibrosis (IPF) or non-specific interstitial pneumonitis (NSIP),with crackles only heard in patients with PPFE who have co-existing lower lobe involvement, this typically being UIP [45]. In those patients with RAS/PPFE after lung transplant, an overall diminishment of breath sounds or wheezing may been heard in patients with RAS/PPFE due to the concomitant presence of BOS [52, 53]. Nail clubbing is less frequently seen in PPFE or RAS/PPFE after lung transplant, compared to that in other chronic lung diseases, with it being present in only 4–25% of patients with PPFE after HSCT [39].

A diagnosis of PPFE is commonly suspected based on the unique findings observed on chest imaging as the presenting symptoms described above are non-specific. Imaging reveals upper lobes pleural thickening with subpleural fibrosis consisting of characteristic bands of fibrous tissue extending from the pleura to the hilum, with the upper lobe fibrosis resulting in the upward retraction of the hilum (**Figure 2**) [43, 45, 49, 52, 53, 71–73]. Pneumothoraces may also be seen on chest imaging at the time of presentation or during the disease course [39, 40, 51–53, 70] with pneumothoraces common in these patients occurring in 25–75% of PPFE patients after HSCT during their illness [39, 40, 51]. This is also true in post-lung transplant patients with PPFE. In the initial description of an upper lobe fibrotic ling disease in lung transplant patients by Konen, et al. 71% of their patients had a pneumothorax [52]. Patients with PPFE are at a particular risk of developing a pneumothorax after undergoing a surgical lung biopsy for diagnosis with these commonly persisting for prolonged periods of time after the procedure [39, 45]. In contrast, pleural effusions are rare in patients with PPFE or RAS/PPFE in the absence of cardiac or renal dysfunction or volume overload. Similar to chest x-ray imaging, chest CT scans more clearly reveal the pleural thickening and fibrotic bands extending from the pleura to the hilum (**Figure 3**). Although predominately an upper lobe process, post HSCT and lung transplant RAS/PPFE does less frequently involve the lower lobes and when involved a third of the patients will have an equal distribution between the upper and lower lobes, particularly later in the course of the disease [41, 45, 46, 53, 74]. The pattern on imaging in the lower lobes is variable compared to that in the upper lobes and can show the typical pleural thickening with fibrous bands extending toward the hilum as seen with upper lobe involvement, but may also show interstitial thickening indicative of interstitial lung disease [40, 45–47, 52, 53, 71]. Pathologically these findings from the lower lobes may be consistent with PPFE but may also show UIP, NSIP or even bronchiolitis obliterans with organizing pneumonia [41, 45–47, 52, 53, 71]. This occurs in 32–75% of all patients with PPFE after HSCT and lung transplant but may also be seen in the idiopathic forms of PPFE [31, 45–47, 52, 53, 71]. Differentiating the presence of UIP (clinically idiopathic pulmonary fibrosis) or NSIP co-existing with PPFE can be challenging. In cases of NSIP and IPF upper lobe findings of fibrotic bands and subpleural thickening on imaging would be atypical and therefore not suggestive of either UIP or NSIP. The only way to definitively diagnose a concomitant interstitial lung disease in the setting of PPFE would be an open lung biopsy. However, as stated above, an open lung biopsy is associated with a significant risk of a prolonged pneumothorax with PPFE and accordingly lung biopsy should be avoided in these patients. The use biomarkers, as will be discussed later, may be clinically helpful in differentiating concomitant interstitial lung disease and PPFE. Although this has not been fully explored, a non-invasive test to diagnose PPFE and exclude other interstitial lung diseases would be of great assistance. Finally, the significance of

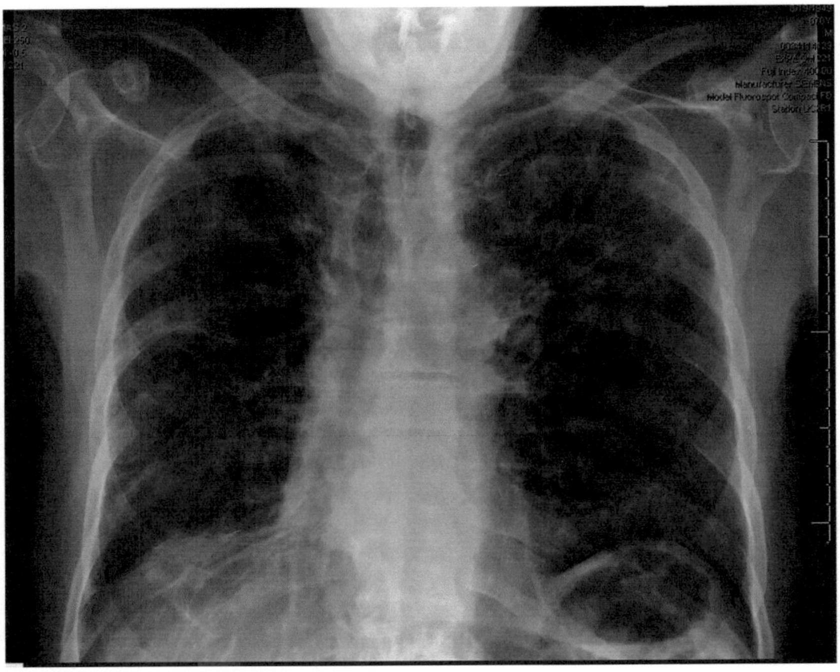

Figure 2.
Chest x-ray of PPFE patient. Note diffuse interstitial changes present and maintenance of normal lung volumes.

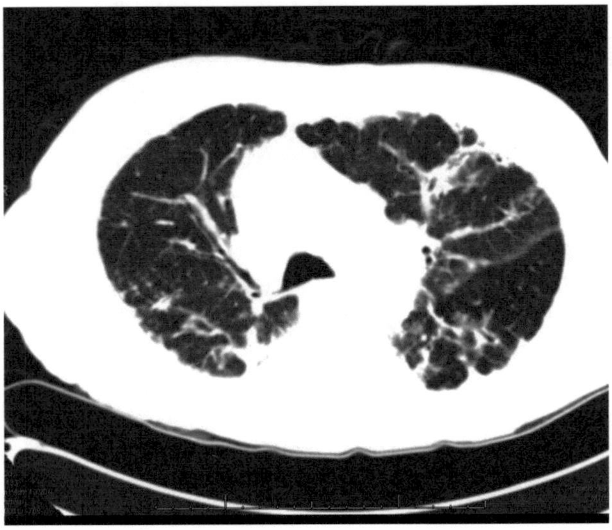

Figure 3.
Corresponding chest CT of patient in ***Figure*** *2. Note subpleural thickening and fibrotic bands radiating toward hilum.*

finding a co-existing interstitial lung disease in patients with post HSCT PPFE or RAS/PPFE after lung transplant, as it relates to etiology and clinical outcomes, is at present not fully known but the presence of lower lobe involvement may influence the clinical course and overall prognosis. The finding of ILD in post lung transplant patients would raise concerns of possible recurrence of the primary disease that led to lung transplantation.

3.5 Pulmonary physiology

Findings on pulmonary function testing performed on patients with PPFE show a significant decline (typically below 60%) in the forced vital capacity (FVC) and an increase in the residual volume to total lung capacity (RV/TLC) ratio [39, 43, 45, 47, 70, 74] with the RV/TLC ratio inversely correlated with the FVC [74]. This RV/TLC ratio of >115% of normal can be useful in differentiating PPFE from the other idiopathic interstitial pneumonias, particularly in those with lower lobe involvement and concerns for a concomitant ILD, as lung biopsy is prohibitive in these patients, as described above [39, 75]. The diffusion capacity is also decreased in PPFE but to a lesser extent than is seen in idiopathic pulmonary fibrosis [39, 45]. Caution in using a decline in FVC in patients who have undergone lung transplant as those patients with RAS/PPFE also commonly have concomitant bronchiolitis obliterans syndrome and therefore mixed disease [48, 49]. Co-existing BOS and RAS occurs in several patients with CLAD after lung transplant with several patients developing BOS followed by RAS [48]. In such a situation the FVC will be decreased with also a decline in the FEV-1/FVC ratio for BOS, whereas in RAS/PPFE the FEV-1/FVC will be increased. In the situation of a decline in FVC but a normal FEV-1/FVC ratio, concomitant BOS and RAS/PPFE must be considered and requires clinical expertise. No detailed algorithm using data from pulmonary function testing has been published to identify patients with combined BOS and RAS/PPFE.

In contrast to the findings on pulmonary function testing, chest imaging, and lung histology with sub-pleural fibrosis and decrease in lung volumes, interestingly exercise capacity is not diminished and oxygen saturation remain normal patients with PPFE, even with exertion, at the time of diagnosis [70]. Further studies need to be performed to determine exercise tolerance and future need for oxygen in these patients long-term. There are several longer-term follow-up studies showing that patients with PPFE after HSCT or PPE/RAS after lung transplant develop progressive disease leading to respiratory failure and the need for supplemental oxygen [39, 40, 47, 52, 53]. Typically repeat pulmonary function tests in most patients show a gradual decrease in the FVC with a corresponding increase in the RV/TLC ratio over time [42, 53, 71, 74]. However, in some patients this change occurs more rapid with a increase in their symptoms and findings of desaturation at rest or with activity [75, 76].

3.6 Challenges with establishing a diagnosis

The initial patients described with post-HSCT PPFE, or upper lobe fibrosis after lung transplant, had a diagnosis confirmed via histologic findings by either lung biopsy or at the time of autopsy [22, 38, 46, 52, 53, 71]. However, patients with PPFE are at high risk for pneumothorax after undergoing lung biopsy, with this pneumothorax potentially persisting for some time after surgery [39, 40, 70, 73]. In addition to a pneumothorax as a complication from a lung biopsy there is a risk for the development of acute respiratory failure due to the presence of co-existing ILD, particularly UIP, and the development of an acute UIP exacerbation [40]. Accordingly, confirmation of PPFE by surgical biopsy should be avoided in these patients. Other forms of lung biopsy (e.g. transbronchial or cryobiopsy via bronchoscope) should also be avoided due the risk for pneumothorax [77, 78]. In addition, the yield from these biopsies techniques are much lower with the risk for complications outweighing the potential diagnostic yield [77, 78]. Recently, several studies have outlined protocols to be used for establishing a diagnosis of PPFE after HSCT in leu of obtaining lung tissue. Early studies focused solely on radiographic imaging for the diagnosis of PPFE [40, 71]. In the study by Reddy et al. radiologic diagnostic criteria were outlined to separate patients into definite, consistent with, or inconsistent with the diagnosis of PPFE with these findings then paired with lung tissue histologic that were similarly graded as definite, consistent with, or inconsistent with PPFE [71]. A limitation of the study by Reddy et al. is that lung tissue was required to confirm the diagnosis of PPFE, which is commonly not present due to current guidelines [71]. However, findings of a correlate between radiographic imaging and histology is extremely useful in establishing a radiographic only diagnosis of PPFE, similar to that commonly now used in multidisciplinary group (MDG) conferences for UIP. Another limitation of this study was that no attempts were made to establish a correlation between clinical symptoms or lung physiology and histologic and chest imaging findings in their patients. Such a study would then mirror the usefulness of MDG conference for the diagnosis of UIP. In a later study, Enomoto, et al. described their approach to the clinical diagnosis of PPFE in a multicenter study by only chest CT imaging utilizing a similar grading system as that used by Reddy et al. [40, 71] wherein their study required radiologic progression as a confirmation of PPFE to avoid including patients with the benign process apical cap disease [40, 71]. A limitation of this study is the requirement for radiologic progression to confirm a diagnosis of PPFE as PPFE in most patients slowly progresses thereby potentially missing patients with PPFE and delaying the diagnosis and possibility for closer follow-up or initiation of treatment and involvement of patients in clinical trials. Finally, Watanabe et al. proposed an algorithm for the diagnosis of PPFE in patients that did or did not undergo a surgical lung biopsy (SLB) with patients placed into diagnostic groups based on their imaging and lung histology, when available [79]. In contrast to other studies, the study by Watanabe et al. used clinical signs and symptoms to generate their algorithm [79]. A definite diagnosis of PPFE was made in those with histologic findings consistent of PPFE in the setting of upper lobe findings of subpleural consolidation and fibrosis on radiographic imaging. However, if lower lobe findings were observed on imaging this required discussion by a MDG to establish a diagnosis. As this study also included clinical data, this study was the first to describe distinct diagnostic groups being radiologically probable PPFE and those with both radiologic and physiologic findings that were probable for PPFE, with the latter group needing respiratory symptoms or respiratory symptoms plus the physiologic abnormalities of a low BMI, decrease in FVC, and an increase in the RV/TLC ratio [79]. This algorithm at present seems to be the optimal way to diagnose PPFE as it only requires available radiologic imaging, clinical findings, and pulmonary function results without the need for disease progression to confirm a diagnosis of PPFE. In contrast to PPFE after HSCT or the idiopathic forms, no detailed studies have been published of diagnosing PPFE in RAS patients after lung transplant.

At present the approach as outlined in the study by Watanabe et al. is now considered to be standard for the diagnosis of PPFE [79]. As an extension to this study, similar to the protocols used in the diagnosis of other IIP's, use of an multidiscipilinary group (MDG) that involves clinicians, radiologists, and pathologists has been suggested as a way to diagnosis PPFE [79, 80]. Use of this approach was outlined in in a review of MDG confirmed cases of PPFE from a nationwide database in Japan examining clinical and radiologic features [80]. We would advocate using the algorithm as outlined by Watanabe et al. in considering a diagnosis of PPFE with inclusion of a MDG to confirm the diagnosis. This will allow for an earlier diagnosis of PPFE and facilitate inclusion of patients in research trials and attempts at new therapeutic strategies. Stressing the importance of using a MDG to diagnose PPFE is that at present, apart from symptoms, lung physiology, and radiographic findings, there are no established body fluid biomarkers to make a diagnosis of PPFE. The lack of such diagnostic biomarkers limits the ability to conclusively make a diagnosis of PPFE and more importantly does not allow for the identification of patients at risk for the rapid progression of PPFE and the corresponding poor prognosis in these patients. The current status of biomarkers in the diagnosis of post-HSCT PPFE and RAS/PPFE after lung transplantation will be discussed below.

3.7 Biomarkers

The availability of biomarkers to assist in the diagnosis of PPFE and RAS/PPFE would be extremely helpful, both in establishing a diagnosis and for the identification of novel therapies. Unfortunately, at present, no such biomarker exists for the definitive diagnose PPFE or RAS/PPFE. The use of biomarkers would be helpful to identify PPFE patients at risk for rapid progression in order to target this group for enrollment in therapeutic clinical trials particularly as the rate of progression and mortality in PPFE and RAS/PPFE is quite variable. Biomarker studies for PPFE and RAS/PPFE have explored the use of urinary desmosines, Krebs von den Lungen-6 (KL6), surfactant protein D (SPD), latent transforming growth factor-β binding protein 4 (LTBP-4), lipocalcin-2, matrix metalloproteinase 9 (MMP-9), and cartilage oligomeric matrix protein (COMP) (**Table 3**) [39, 61–65, 80–87]. Early studies examining these biomarkers suggest that they may be helpful in the diagnosis of PPFE and RAS/PPFE and/or their prognosis and clinical outcomes, however further

Biomarkers for PPFE
Desmosine
Increased levels in PPFE; discriminatory for PPFE vs. COPD vs. IPF
Krebs von den Lungen-6 (KL-6)
Higher in PPFE vs. IPF
Increased levels in CLAD (BOS/RAS) vs. non-CLAD post lung transplant
May be helpful for prognostics
Cartilage oligomeric protein (COMP)
Potentially predictive for development of RAS
Lipocalcin-2
May differentiate RAS vs. BOS in CLAD patients
Matrix metalloproteinase 9 (MMP9)
Potentially predictive for development of BOS
Correlates with decline in lung function
Latent transforming growth factor-β binding protein 4 (LTB4)
Increased levels in PPFE vs. IPF
Higher levels correlate with lung function decline
Surfactant protein D
Increased levels in PPFE

Table 3.
The above is a list of the current biomarkers that have been examined for the diagnosis and management of PPFE.

studies are necessary to confirm these preliminary studies. As discussed below, the potential use of biomarkers in PPFE has focused on those with idiopathic PPFE, but hope would be that these results could be extended to patients with PPFE from defined causes, including post_HSCT and RAS/PPFE. At present, no study has examined biomarkers in patients specifically with post-HSCT PPFE. In contrast, the studies described below in patients with RAS are specific to that diagnosis but not specifically to RAS/PPFE.

Desmosines are breakdown products of elastase. As patients with PPFE have active lung fibrosis it was hypothesized that urinary levels of desmosines would be higher in PPFE patients [82]. In addition, as fibrosis rates are higher in patients with PPFE compared to IPF, an elevation in desmosines breakdown products may be useful in differentiating between PPFE and IPF [82]. This possibility was explored in a study measuring urinary desmosine levels in patients with biopsy proven PPFE compared to levels in patients with idiopathic pulmonary fibrosis (IPF), chronic obstructive disease (COPD), or controls [82]. Findings from this study showed that urinary desmosines levels were significantly higher in PPFE patients compared to control patients and that they were also higher in those with chronic obstructive pulmonary disease (COPD). Furthermore desmosines levels were higher in those with PPFE compared to IPF and that levels were able to discriminate between the diagnosis of PPFE and IPF. In contrast, urinary desmosine levels did not correlate with clinical parameters (e.g. BMI), physiology(pulmonary function testing, PaO_2, or 6 minute walk distance), or disease severity [82]. Accordingly, this does allow for the use of urinary desmosines in a multidisciplinary approach to the diagnosis of PPFE at this time. As only a single time point was examined in this study, it is not clear if urinary desmosines levels are useful longitudinally to determine disease progression, morbidity, or prognosis. Measurements of urinary desmosines may be clinically useful at present to differentiate between PPFE and IPF in patients with lower lobe involvement or imaging findings that are suggestive of IPF. Further studies are necessary to determine the role of urinary desmosines in the diagnosis of PPFE and if they are useful in the diagnosis of RAS/PPFE, wherein they have not been examined.

Levels of KL-6 have been shown to be useful in the diagnosis of PPFE, with the ability to differentiate PPFE from other forms of idiopathic interstitial pneumonias (IIP), and have also been beneficial in the diagnosis of RAS/PPFE and the ability to differentiate between BOS and RAS in patients with CLAD [63, 65, 82, 86, 87]. In addition, KL-6 levels also appear to be helpful for prognostics. Levels of KL-6 between those with PPFE and IPF were examined by Oyama et al. and it was found that levels of KL-6 were significantly higher in IPF patients compared to those with PPFE although no potential correlation between KL-6 levels and clinical characteristics or physiologic variables in the PPFE group were explored [82]. In a later study by Ishii et al. [80] this specific question was addressed. Results from that study showed that PPFE patients with an elevated level of KL-6 had a decreased median survival (24 months shorter) over a 5 year follow-up period than those with KL-6 levels under 600 U/ml [80]. These findings were replicated by Kinoshita et al. wherein patients with KL-6 levels over 550 U/ml had an overall poorer prognosis [83]. Similarly, in studying systemic sclerosis patients with PPFE, d'Alessandro et al. found that patients with a significant decline in their FVC and FEV-1, indicative of clinical progression, also had increasing serum KL-6 levels [81]. In that study KL-6 levels were measured serially over a 6 year time frame which increased the study's clinical relevance. Although these studies would suggest a role for KL-6 in the diagnosis and management of PPFE, a small study by Sato et al. found no difference in KL-6 levels in PPFE patients [84]. Accordingly, further investigation is necessary to establish a role of KL-6 in the diagnosis or management of idiopathic and secondary PPFE.

Regarding the use of KL-6 in the diagnosis of RAS/PPFE after lung transplantation, levels of KL-6 in the serum and bronchoalveolar lavage fluid have been examined in patients with CLAD to determine both the diagnosis of CLAD and to differentiate those with BOS from those with RAS/PPFE. The initial study by Walter et al. examined if serum KL-6 levels could differentiate post lung transplant patients with BOS versus transplant patients without BOS as well as from normal controls [86]. KL-6 were significantly increased in post lung transplant patients with BOS compared to those without BOS and to normal controls with mean levels over 2 fold higher whereas the levels in post lung transplant patients without BOS did not significantly differ compared to healthy controls. This study was performed prior to the description of RAS as a post lung transplant complication and therefore patients with RAS may have been included in the BOS group and therefore results cannot be directly extended to RAS/PPFE. Other limitations of this study were the small sample size, that only a single time point was examined, and there was no discussion regarding the timing of blood collection as it relates to the time after lung transplantation. Similar findings were observed by Ohshimo et al. when they examined serum KL-6 levels in post lung transplant patients with BOS compared to those without BOS as well as healthy controls [87]. A strength of this study is that serial serum KL-6 levels were obtained at the time patients underwent bronchoscopy for clinical indications. Again, serum KL-6 levels were significantly increased in post lung transplant patients with BOS compared to those without BOS and to healthy controls. Mean KL-6 levels were over two fold higher in BOS patients compared to healthy controls and almost two fold higher when compared to patients without BOS. The study did not discuss if KL-6 levels changed over time in the groups. Importantly this studied compared the KL-6 levels between the two CLAD subtypes, BOS and RAS. The levels of KL-6 were significantly increased in RAS patients compared to those with BOS with mean values over two times higher. KL-6 levels also correlated with the decline in FEV-1in BOS subjects, thereby providing a clinical relevance to their study. Finally, Berastegui et al. asked the question if KL-6 levels in bronchoalveolar lavage fluid would be helpful in diagnosing CLAD, and in particular RAS [63]. Interestingly in this study there was no significant difference in serum KL-6 levels between post lung transplant patients with BOS and those that were stable after transplant and to healthy controls. However, similar to the results described above, serum KL-6 levels in RAS patients were significantly increased compared to lung transplant patients without CLAD and to healthy controls with mean serum KL-6 levels over three times higher than these other groups. In contrast, levels of KL-6 in the bronchoalveolar lavage fluid did not differ between the groups. Similar to the results by Ohshimo et al., serum KL-6 levels correlated with lung function testing, specifically the forced vital capacity (FVC), where higher serum KL-6 levels correlated with a decrease in FVC levels [63, 87].

Other biomarkers examined to diagnose CLAD and to differentiate BOS from RAS include cartilage oligomeric matric protein (COMP), Lipocalcin-2, and matrix metalloproteinase 9 (MMP9) [61, 64–66]. A retrospective study by Novo et al. examined if serial measurements of COMP could predict the later development of CLAD, including BOS and RAS [66]. Levels of COMP were higher at 3 months prior to the development of RAS, whereas COMP levels were not significantly different when comparing patients with CLAD as a whole to transplant patients that did not develop CLAD [66]. This suggests that COMP may be useful to differentiate RAS from BOS in CLAD patients. Patients with PPFE were not highlighted in this study. Similarly lipocalcin-2 levels were found to be elevated in patients with RAS in comparison to BOS [64]. Staining for lipocalcin 2 was present in distal airways and alveolar walls, where RAS is thought to originate [64]. Metalloproteinase 9 (MMP-9) has been linked to fibrotic diseases and has been studied as a biomarker for IPF. As fibrosis is an underlying cause for the symptoms and pathologic findings in the two types of CLAD, BOS (airway) and RAS (alveoli and interstitium), levels of MMP-9 have been examined to determine if they can diagnose CLAD as well as be a predictor for its occurrence [48, 86, 88, 89]. Beeh et al. examined MMP-9 levels in sputum from lung transplant patients and found that levels were higher in lung transplant patients compared to healthy controls with the highest levels seen in those diagnosed with BOS [88]. Similar findings were observed by Hubner et al. that found the ratio of MMP-9 to tissue inhibitor of MMPs (TIMP-1) was higher in lung transplant patients with BOS [89]. Importantly there was a correlation of sputum MMP-9: TIMP-1 ratios to spirometric values and in particular FEV-1. Finally, Pain et al. examined the use of serum MMP-9 levels as a predictor for the onset of BOS [61]. MMP-9 levels were serially measured for 18 months prior to the onset of CLAD. An increase in MMP-9 levels 12 months prior to the onset of CLAD predicted its occurrence with a stronger association with BOS than with RAS. Again, these studies assessed the levels of MMP-9 in patients with BOS, and not always specifically to RAS, without specific mention of PPFE.

Ongoing elastogenesis has been suggested to correlate with the levels of LTBP-4 and accordingly levels of LTB4 have also been explored as a biomarker for the diagnosis of PPFE [83]. Kinoshita et al. in their study measured LTBP-4 levels in both lung tissue and in serum from patients with either lung biopsy confirmed PPFE or those that were clinically diagnosed PPFE with these levels compared to those from healthy controls. Serum levels of LTBP-4 in PPFE patients were significantly higher than in controls and furthermore were 50% higher compared to patients with IPF [83]. Similar results were found for LTBP-4 levels in the lung, wherein PPFE patients had levels 2 fold higher than those with IPF [83]. Interestingly, levels of LTBP-4 in the serum of IPF patients who had co-existing upper lobe PPFE had higher levels compared to IPF patients without co-existing PPFE. Taken together this suggests that LTBP-4 may be a more specific biomarker for PPFE. This study also examined for a potential correlation between clinical parameters and survival with LTBP-4 levels with findings that a significant decline in FVC or the RV/TLC ratio trended with higher LTBP-4 levels in the serum. Higher LTBP-4 levels were associated with a 20% lower survival rate compared to those with normal LTBP-4 levels [83]. Upon comparison of the relative value between KL-6 and LTBP-4 in determining the diagnosis of PPFE versus IPF, levels of KL-6 are more useful for the diagnosis of IPF wherein LTBP-4 levels are useful in the diagnosis as well as management of PPFE [83]. Similar to the study discussed above of KL-6 levels, a limitation of the study is that only a one time measurement of serum LTBP-4 was assessed. Future studies examining serial LTBF-4 measurements would be helpful to determine if levels of LTB-4 can predict PPFE progression rate and prognosis. To date, LTBF-4 has not been examined as a biomarker in RAS/PPFE after lung transplantation.

Levels of surfactant protein D (SPD) have also been examined in PPFE patients to determine its use as a potential biomarker [40, 84, 85, 90, 91]. Several small studies found that SPD levels are increased in PPFE, however levels of SPD did not correlate to baseline physiologic values or patient demographics. Levels of SPD, in a cluster analysis study designed to identify PPFE prognostic factors, did trend with mortality rates that were highest [90]. Additional studies using larger patient cohorts are needed define a potential role for SPD levels in the diagnosis and management of PPFE and in particular if SPD levels over time identifies those patients with a higher risk for rapid progression of disease or a decrease in survival rate. Additional studies are also needed to examine its potential role in RAS/PPFE.

The above studies examining potential biomarkers in PPFE were mostly done in patients with the idiopathic form of the disease and not those specific to post-HSCT or lung transplantation. Pathologic findings from lung tissue obtained by biopsy and autopsy are similar for patients with an identified etiology for PPFE (post-HSCT patients or lung transplant patients with RAS/PPFE) and idiopathic PPFE suggesting that the above described biomarkers may also be helpful in the diagnosis and management PPFE that occurs after HSCT or in RAS/PPFE after lung transplantation.

3.8 Treatment, clinical course, and prognosis

To date no pharmacologic treatment for PPFE after HSCT or for RAS/PPFE in lung transplant patients has been identified to improve symptoms or to slow or reverse the progression of disease. In regards to post-HSCT patients, several case series describe patients that were treated with corticosteroids, however such treatment was not beneficial in slowing down the disease process or changing outcomes [39, 42, 45, 51, 70]. Similarly, as for HSCT patients the initiation, or increase in dose, of other immunosuppressants, such as cyclosporin, cyclophosphamide, mycophenolate, sirolimus, or tacrolimus has been tried in lung transplant patients but has not been shown to slow down or reverse the disease [38, 50, 54]. Other adjunctive treatments, including N-acetylcysteine and azithromycin, have been tried but there are no reports of a consistent response to these treatments [39, 42, 70]. That being said, for lung transplant patients azithromycin has been shown to be effective in the treatment of neutrophil reversible allograft dysfunction, a distinct entity apart from RAS with its own pathophysiology, but has not been effective in the treatment of RAS [38, 50]. Photophoresis therapy has been tried in lung transplant patients with RAS/PPFE but similar to other treatments described above has not been shown to be effective, although it may be helpful in those with strictly BOS [92, 93]. Recently, use of nintedanib and pirfenidone has been described in a small series of patients with either idiopathic or secondary PPFE [37, 91] and in case reports after lung transplant in those with RAS/PPFE [94, 95]. In the study by Nasser et al. the decline in FVC was less in those that received nintedanib compared to placebo, however the upper lobe volume loss determined by CT measurements did not differ over time between groups [38, 91]. In the case report by Pluchart et al. regarding the use of nintedanib in a post-lung transplant patient, there was no clinical change after 4 months of treatment with treatment eventually discontinued due to adverse effects [95]. For pirfenidone, in the case report by Sato et al., their patient had stable pulmonary function tests after initiation of pirfenidone, however this patient had mixed PPFE and UIP, as confirmed by open lung biopsy, so it is unclear if the PPFE responded to pirfenidone or just the UIP [94]. In regards to the pharmacologic treatment for PPFE, future studies are necessary to identify biomarkers and pathophysiologic mechanism in order to design novel pharmacologic approaches for the treatment of PPFE.

For those with progressive disease and respiratory failure, the only treatment option at present is lung transplantation [39, 47, 70, 96–98]. To date only 50 patients have been described that have undergone lung transplantation for PPFE, with most of these patients described in case reports or small case series [96–98]. Overall these studies describe the unique difficulties in performing lung transplants in PPFE and

RAS/PPFE patients including pleural and chest wall adhesions, the flat thorax commonly seen, and the low body mass index (BMI). In the single center study by Faccioli et al. the median survival after lung transplant for PPFE patients was 24.5 months which is significantly decreased compared to the lung transplant patients as a whole who currently have a median survival of 62.5 months [98]. This is in contrast to the study by Shiya et al. that showed that mortality after lung transplant in patients with PPFE did not differ compared to those with ILD [99]. Larger studies are necessary to fully understand the role of lung transplant as a treatment for PPFE as a whole. However, what does seem clear from the literature is that patients with secondary PPFE to do clinically worse after lung transplant compared to those with the idiopathic form with survival times of around only 8 months [98].

The diagnosis of PPFE is associated with a poor prognosis after HSCT with 5 year survival rates estimated at 23.3–58.9%, although the median survival rate is 11.8 years [39, 40, 71, 83]. For patients with RAS/PPFE after lung transplant, the two studies initially describing PPFE in lung transplant patients gave no specific mention of life expectancy in their patients [49, 52]. Although no direct study on mortality after lung transplant in those with RAS with predominately PPFE has been performed, the overall survival after development of RAS is 6–18 months, suggesting a poorer prognosis for PPFE after lung transplant than after HSCT [54]. Interestingly, after either HSCT or lung transplantation two clinical scenarios have been described in the course of PPFE suggesting a common mechanism and pathophysiology. The two courses are either of a slow progression of disease over several months to years or a more precipitous decline, with the former being the clinical course that typically occurs [45, 74, 75, 97]. Currently there are no identified risk factors or clinical features to accurately predict the clinical course of an individual patient, nor are there known precipitants that causes transition from a slow progressive disease and induces a rapid progression or acute decompensation of the disease process. Progression of PPFE is typically manifested by progressive fibrosis and continued upper lobe volume loss, onset of radiographic changes in the mid and lower lung fields, continued weight loss and a decreasing BMI, further flattening of the thoracic cage with impairment of respiratory mechanics, an increase in shortness of breath and dyspnea on exertion, and acute respiratory failure [45, 53, 74, 79, 99]. Physiologically there is a continued decline in the FVC and radiographically pneumothoraces may be observed in addition to the signs of increased fibrosis [45, 52, 74, 79, 99]. This progression in volume loss was well outlined in the case series by Konen et al. where progressive lung changes were seen during serial yearly chest CT reviews over a greater than 4 year time frame [53]. Specifically in regards to radiographic changes, findings of lower lobe involvement and/or the co-existing interstitial lung disease, has been associated with a rapid progression in the disease course as well as shorter survival times [100]. It is unclear if this represents solely a progression of PPFE or the development of a secondary interstitial lung disease. Recently, studies in post HSCT patients have described scoring systems to assist in determining the prognosis of individuals with PPFE. Unfortunately no such scoring system is available for post lung transplant patients with RAS/PPFE after lung transplantation. The gender-age-physiology (GAP) model is a prognostic tool used for idiopathic pulmonary fibrosis patients [80]. This model was evaluated for patients with PPFE after HSCT by Shioya et al. and showed that those with a higher GAP score had a worse prognosis [99]. Kinoshita et al. recently published a PPFE prognostic model using variables shown to be significant in post-HSCT PPFE patients [41]. By examining data from two large patient cohorts with PPFE and using a multivariate Cox regression model they were able to identify 4 variables that predicted mortality in PPFE. Variables found to be important included forced vital capacity, history of pneumothorax, findings of lower lobe interstitial lung disease, and serum KL-6 levels [83]. A point system was derived using these four variables with three patient groups identified predicting survival based on the total score. The above type of studies are necessary but require further development, expansion, and refinement to allow scoring systems to prognosticate patients' expected outcomes and clinical course and when attempt treatment or enrollment in clinical treatment trials.

Author details

Pat Arndt
Division of Pulmonary, Critical Care, Allergy, and Sleep Medicine, University of Minnesota, Minneapolis, MN, United States

*Address all correspondence to: arndt108@umn.edu

References

[1] Wanko S, Broadwater G, Folz R, Chao N. Diffuse alveolar hemorrhage: Retrospective review of clinical outcomes in allogeneic transplant recipients treated with aminocaproic acid. Biology of Blood and Marrow Transplantation. 2006;**12**:949-953

[2] Yanik G, Hellerstedt B, Custer J, Hutchinson R, Kwon D, et al. Etanercept (Enbrel) administration for idiopathic pneumonia syndrome after allogeneic hematopoietic stem cell transplantation. Biology of Blood and Marrow Transplantation. 2002;**8**:395-400

[3] Valapour M, Lehr C, Schladt D, et al. OPTN/SRTR. Annual data report lung. Scientific registry of transplant recipients. 2021

[4] Van der Mark S, Hoek R, Hellemons M. Developments in lung transplantation over the last decade. European Respiratory Review. 2020;**29**:190132

[5] Rathi NK, Tanner AR, Dinh A, Dong W, Feng L, et al. Low-, medium-, or high-dose steroids with or without aminocaproic acid in adult hematopoietic SCT patients with diffuse alveolar hemorrhage. Bone Marrow Transplantation. 2015;**50**:420-426

[6] Holm AM, Riise GC, Hansson L, Brinch L, Bjørtuft O, et al. Lung transplantation for bronchiolitis obliterans syndrome after Allo-SCT. Bone Marrow Transplantation. 2013;**48**:703-707

[7] Arndt A, Boffa D. Pleural space complications associated with lung transplantation. Thoracic Surgery Clinics. 2015;**25**:87-95

[8] Tang A, Siddiqui H, Thuita L, et al. Natural history of pleural complications after lung transplantation. The Annals of Thoracic Surgery. 2021;**111**:407-415

[9] Joean O, Kayser M, Valtin C, et al. Characteristics and clinical implications of pleural effusions after lung transplantation: A retrospective analysis of 195 thoracentesis in 113 patients. Clinical Transplantation. 2021;**35**:e14267

[10] Martino R, Porras RP, Rabella N. Prospective study of the incidence, clinical features, and outcome of symptomatic upper and lower respiratory tract infections by respiratory viruses in adult recipients of hematopoietic stem cell transplants for hematologic malignancies. Biology of Blood and Marrow Transplantation. 2005;**11**:781-796

[11] Seo S, Renaud C, Kuypers JM, Chiu CY, Huang ML, et al. Idiopathic pneumonia syndrome after hematopoietic cell transplantation: Evidence of occult infectious etiologies. Blood. 2015;**125**:3789-3797

[12] Neofytos D, Horn D, Anaissie E, Steinbach W, Olyaei A, et al. Epidemiology and outcomes of invasive fungal infection in adult hematopoietic stem cell transplant recipients; analysis of multicenter prospective antifungal therapy (PATH) alliance registry. Clinical Infectious Diseases. 2009;**48**:265-273

[13] Auberger J, Lass-Flörl C, Ulmer H, Nogler-Semenitz E, Clausen J, et al. Significant alterations in the epidemiology and treatment outcome of invasive fungal infections in patients with hematological malignancies. International Journal of Hematology. 2008;**88**:508-515

[14] Dettori M, Riccardi N, Canetti D, et al. Infections in lung transplanted patients: A review. Pulmonology. DOI: S2531-0437(22)00118-0

[15] Trachuk P, Bartash R, Abbasi M, et al. Infectious complications in lung transplant recipients. Lung. 2020;**198**:879-887

[16] Ferrer J, Roldan J, Roman A, et al. Acute and chonic pleural complications in lung transplantation. The Journal of Heart and Lung Transplantation. 2003;**22**:1217-1225

[17] Shitrit D, Izbicki G, Fink G, et al. Late postoperative pleural effusion following lung transplantation: Characteristics and clinical implications. European Journal of Cardio-Thoracic Surgery. 2003;**23**:494-496

[18] Modi D, Jang H, Kim S, Deol A, Ayash L, et al. Incidence, etiology, and outcome of pleural effusions in allogeneic hematopoietic stem cell transplantation. American Journal of Hematology. 2016;**91**:E341-E347

[19] Leonard JT, Newell LF, Meyers G, Hayes-Lattin B, Gajewski J, et al. Chronic GvHD-associated serositis and pericarditis. Bone Marrow Transplantation. 2015;**50**:1098-1104

[20] Mohamedaly O, Mulroney C, Makani S. Serositis as a rare pulmonary manifestation of chronic graft-versus-host disease. Chest. 2013;**144**(4):489A-489B

[21] Nguyen A, Bashoura L, Jimenez C, Morice R, Ost D, Eapen G, et al. Characteristics of pleural effusions in patients after hematopoietic stem cell transplantation. Chest. 2010;**138**(4):812A

[22] Von der Thusen J, Hansell D, Tominaga M, et al. Pleuroparenchymal fibroelastosis in patients with pulmonary disease secondary to bone marrow transplantation. Modern Pathology. 2011;**24**:1633-1639

[23] Herridge MS, de Hoyos AL, Chapoarro C, et al. Pleural complications in lung transplant recipients. The Journal of Thoracic and Cardiovascular Surgery. 1995;**110**:22-26

[24] Leard L. Pleural complications in lung transplantation. UpToDate September 2023

[25] Hochberg MC. Updating the American College of Rheumatology revised criteria for the classification of systemic lupus erythematosus. Arthritis and Rheumatism. 1997;**40**:1725

[26] Dobbie JW. Serositis: Comparative analysis of histological findings and pathogenetic mechanisms in nonbacterial serosal inflammation. Peritoneal Dialysis International. 1993;**13**(4):256-269

[27] Man BL, Mok CC. Serositis related to systemic lupus erythematosus: Prevalence and outcome. Lupus. 2005;**14**:822-826

[28] Yan L, Rui-Xue L, Hai-Feng P, Dong-Qing Y. The prevalence and risk factors for serositis in patients with systemic lupus erythematosus: A cross-sectional study. Rheumatology International. 2017;**37**(2):305-311

[29] Abu-Hijleh M, Evans S. Pleuropericarditis in a patient with inflammatory bowel disease: A case presentation and review of the literature. Lung. 2010;**188**:505-510

[30] Norkin M, Ratanatharathorn V, Ayash L, Abidi M, Al-Kadhimi Z, Lum L, et al. Large pericardial effusion as a complication in adults undergoing SCT. Bone Marrow Transplantation. 2010;**46**(10):1353-1356

[31] Liu Y, Gau J, Hong Y, Yu Y, Hsiao L, Liu J, et al. Large pericardial effusion as a life-threatening complication after hematopoietic stem cell transplantation—Association with

chronic GVHD in late-onset adult patients. Annals of Hematology. 2012;**91**(12):1953-1958

[32] Seber A, Khan S, Kersey J. Unexplained effusions: Association with allogenic bone marrow transplantation and acute or chronic graft-versus-host disease. Bone Marrow Transplantation. 1996;**17**(2):207-211

[33] Nagler A, Rocha V, Labopin M, Unal A, Ben Othman T, Campos A, et al. Allogeneic hematopoietic stem-cell transplantation for acute myeloid leukemia in remission: Comparison of intravenous busulfan plus cyclophosphamide (Cy) versus total-body irradiation plus cy as conditioning regimen—A report from the acute Leukemia working Party of the European Group for blood and marrow transplantation. Journal of Clinical Oncology. 2013;**31**(28):3549-3556

[34] Cavet J, Lennard A, Gascoigne A, Finney R, Lucraft H, Richardson C, et al. Constrictive pericarditis post allogeneic bone marrow transplant for Philadelphia-positive acute lymphoblastic leukemia. Bone Marrow Transplantation. 2000;**25**(5):571-573

[35] Ballal P, Arndt P, Twaddell. Pleurodesis: A novel treatment option for refractory chronic graft versus host disease associated serositis. Chest. 2017;**532A**

[36] Travis WD, Costabel U, Hansell DM, et al. ATS/ERS committee on idiopathic interstitial pneumonias. An official American Thoracic Society/European Respiratory Society statement: Update of the international multidisciplinary classification of the idiopathic interstitial pneumonias. American Journal of Respiratory and Critical Care Medicine. 2013;**188**:733-748

[37] Amitani R, Niimi A, Kuse F. Idiopoahtic pulmonary upper lobe fibrosis (IPUF). Kokyu. 1992;**11**:693-639

[38] Frankel SK, Cool CD, Lynch BKK. Idiopathic pleuroparenchymal fibroelastosis: Description of a novel clinicopathologic entity. Chest. 2004;**126**:2007-2013

[39] Ricoy J, Suarwez-Antelo J, Antunez J, et al. Pleuroparenchymal fibroelastosis: Clinical, radiological, and histopathological features. Respiratory Medicine. 2022;**191**:106437

[40] Enomoto Y, Nakamura Y, Satake Y, et al. Clinical diagnosis of idiopathic pleuroparanchymal fibroelastosis: A retrospective multicenter study. Respiratory Medicine. 2017;**133**:1-5

[41] Kinoshita Y, Ikeda T, Muyamura T, et al. A proposed prognostic prediction score for pleuroparenchymal fibroelastosis. Respiratory Research. 2021;**22**:215-223

[42] Mariani F, Gatti B, Rocca A, et al. Pleuroparenchymal fibroelastosis: The prevalence of secondary forms in hematopoietic stem cell and lung transplantation recipients. Diagnostic and Interventional Radiology. 2016;**22**:400-406

[43] Namkoong H, Ishii M, Mori T, et al. Clinical and radiological characteristics of patients with lated-onset severe restrictive lung defect after hematopoietic stem cell transplantation. BMC Pulmonary Medicine. 2017;**17**:123-131

[44] Meignin V, Thivolet-Bejui F, Kambouchner M, et al. Lung histopathology of non-infectious pulmonary complications after allogeneic hematopoietic stem cell transplantation. Histopathology. 2018;**73**:832-842

[45] Chua F, Desai S, Nicholson A, et al. Pleureoparenchymal fibroelastosis: A review of clinical, radiological, and

pathological characteristics. Annals of the American Thoracic Society. 2019;**16**:1351-1359

[46] Takeuchi Y, Miyagawa-Hayashino A, Chen F, et al. Pleuroparenchymal fibroelastosis and non-specific interstitial pneumonia: Frequent pulmonary sequelae of haematopoietic stem cell transplantation. Histopathology. 2015;**66**:536-544

[47] Bondeelle L, Gras J, Michonneau D, et al. Pleuroparenchymal fibroelastosis after allogeneic hematopoietic stem cell transplantation. Bone Marrow Transplantation. 2020;**55**:982-986

[48] Glanville A, Vedrleden G, Todd J, et al. Chronic lung allograft dysfunction: Definition and update of restrictive allograft syndrome – A consensus report from the pulmonary council of ISHLT. The Journal of Heart and Lung Transplantation. 2019;**38**:484-492

[49] Ofek E, Sato M, Saito T, et al. Restrictive allograft syndrome post lung transplantation is characterized by pleuroparnchymal fibroelastosis. Modern Pathology. 2013;**26**:350-356

[50] Venado A, Kukreja J, Greenland J. Chronic lung allograft dysfunction. Thoracic Surgery Clinics. 2022;**32**:231-242

[51] Higo H, Miyahara N, Taniguchi A, et al. Cause of pleuroparenchymal fibroelastosis following allogeneic hematopoietic stem cell transplantation. Respiratory Investigation. 2019;**57**:321-324

[52] Konen E, Weisbrod G, Pakhale S, et al. Fibrosis of the upper lobes: A newly identified late-onset complication after lung transplantation? AJR. 2003;**181**:1539-1543

[53] Pakhale S, Hadjiliadis D, Howell D, et al. Upper lobe fibrosis: A novel manifestation of chronic allograft dysfunction in lung transplantation. International Society for Heart and Lung Transplantation. 2005;**24**:1260-1268

[54] Klouda T, Vargas S, Midyat L. Restrictive allograft syndrome after lung transplantation. Pediatric Transplantation. 2021;**25**:e14000

[55] Beynat-Mouterde C, Beltramo G, Lezmi G, et al. Pleuroparenchymal fibroelastosis as a late complication of chemotherapy agents. The European Respiratory Journal. 2014;**44**:523-527

[56] Yamamoto Y, Tsujino K, Kuge T, et al. Pleuroparenchymal fibroelastosis un Mycobacterium avian complex pulmonary disease: Clinical characteristics and prognostic impact. European Respiratory Journal. 2021;7:00765

[57] Aonoi Y, Hozumi H, Kono M, et al. Prognostic significance of radiological pleuroparenchymal fibroelastosis in Mycobacterium avium complex lung disease: A multicentre restrospective cohort study. Thorax. 2023;**78**(8):825-834

[58] Sato M, Hwang D, Ohmri-Matsudas K, et al. Revisiting the pathologic findings of diffuse alveolar damage after lug transplantation. The Journal of Heart and Lung Transplantation. 2012;**31**(4):354-363

[59] Shino M, Weigt S, Li N, et al. CXCR3 ligands are associated with the continuum of diffuse alveolar damage to chronic lung allograft dysfunction. American Journal of Respiratory and Critical Care Medicine. 2013;**188**:1117-1125

[60] Verleden SE, Ruttens D, Vos R, et al. Differential cytokine chemokine and growth factor expression in phenotypes of chronic allograft dysfunction. Transplantation. 2015;**99**:86-93

[61] Pain M, Royer P-J, Loy J, Girardeau A, et al. T cells promote bronchial epithelial cell secretion of matrix metalloproteinase-9 via a C-C chemokine receptor type 2 pathway: Implications for chronic lung allograge dysfunction. American Journal of Transplantation. 2017;**17**:1502-1514

[62] Levy L, Tigert A, Huszti EW, et al. Epithelial cell death markers in bronchoalveolar lavage correlates with chronic lung allograft dysfunction subtypes and survival in lung transplant recipients – A single-center retrospective cohort study. Transplant International. 2019;**32**:965-973

[63] Berastegui C, Gomez-Olles S, Mendoza-VAlderrey A, et al. Use of serum KL-6 level for detecting patients with restrictive allograft syndrome after lung transplantation. PlosOne. 2020

[64] Veraar C, Kliman J, Benazzo A, et al. Potential novel biomarkers for chronic lung allograft dysfunction and azithromycin responsive allograft dysfunction. Scientific Reports. 2021;**11**:6799-6811

[65] Van der Ploeg E, Melgert B, Burgess J, et al. The potential of biomarkers of fibrosis in chronic lung allograft syndrome. Transplantation Reviews. 2021;**35**:100626

[66] Novo M, Westin J, Andersson LM, et al. COMP: A potential early biomarker of RAS after lung transplantation. Transplantation direct. 2021;**e730**

[67] Montero M, Osdadolor T, Khiroya R, et al. Restrictive allograft syndrome and idiopathic pleuroparenchymal fibroelastosis: Do they really have the same histology. Histopathology. 2017;**70**:1107-1111

[68] Todd J, Christie J, Palmer S. Update in lung transplantation 2013. AJRCCM. 2014;**190**:19-24

[69] Verleden SE, Vanaudenaerde BM, Emonds MP, et al. Donor-specific and -nonspecific HLA antibodies and outcome post lung transplantation. The European Respiratory Journal. 2017;**50**(5)

[70] Bonifazi M, Montero A, Benzoni E. Idiopathic pleuroparenchymal fibroelastosis. Current Pulmonology Reports. 2017;**6**:9-15

[71] Reddy T, Tominaga M, Hansell D, et al. Pleuroparenchymal fibroelastosis: A spectrum of histopathological and imaging phenotypes. The European Respiratory Journal. 2012;**40**:377-385

[72] Glanville A, Benden C, Bergeron A, et al. Bronchiolitis obliterans syndrome after lung of hematopoietic stem cell transplantation: Current management and future directions. ERJ Open Research. 2022;**8**:00185

[73] Cottin V, Si-Mohamed S, Diesler R, et al. Pleuroparenchymal fibroelastosis. Current Opinion in Pulmonary Medicine. 2021;**28**:432-440

[74] Yoshida Y, Nagata N, Tsurutua N, et al. Heterogeneous clinical features in patients with pulmonary fibrosis showing histology of pleuroparenchymal fibroelastosis. Respiratory Investigation. 2016;**54**:162-169

[75] Watanabe K, Nagata N, Kitasato Y, et al. Rapid decrease in forced vital capacity in patients with idiopathic pulmonary upper lobe fibrosis. Respiratory Investigation. 2012;**50**:88-97

[76] Murakami Y, Sakamoto K, Okumura Y, et al. Acute exacerbation of pleuroparanchymal fibroelastosis secondary to allogeneic hematopoietic stem cell transplantation. Internal Medicine. 2020;**59**:2737-2743

[77] Hakami A, Zwartkruis E, Radonic E, et al. Transbronchial cryobiopsy for

diagnosis of pleuroparenchymal fibroelastosis. Respiratory Medicine Case Reports. 2020;**31**:101164

[78] Kushima H, Hidaka K, Ishii H, et al. Two cases of pleuroparenchymal fibroelastosis diagnosed with transbronchial biopsy. Respiratory Medicine Case Reports. 2016;**19**:71-73

[79] Watanabe K, Ishii H, Kiyomi F, et al. Criteria for the diagnosis of idiopathic pleuroparenchymal fibroelastosis: A proposal. Respiratory Investigation. 2019;**57**:312-320

[80] Ishii H, Watanabe K, Kushima H, et al. Pleuroparenchymal fibroelastosis diagnosed by multidisciplinary discussions in Japan. Respiratory Medicine. 2018;**141**:190197. Online: 0226488

[81] d'Alessandro M, Bellisia F, Bergantini L, et al. Prognostic role of KL-6 in SSc-ILD patients with pleuroparenchymal fibroelastosis. European Journal of Clinical Investigation. 2021;**51**:e13543

[82] Oyama Y, Enomoto N, Suzuki Y, et al. Evaluation of urinary desmosines as a noninvasive diagnostic biomarker in patients with idiopathic pleuroparenchymal fibroelastosis (PPFE). Respiratory Medicine. 2017;**123**:63-70

[83] Kinoshita Y, Ikeda T, Kushima H, et al. Serum latent transforming growth factor-b binding protein 4 as a novel biomarker for idiopathic pleuroparenchymal fibroelastosixs. Respiratory Medicine. 2020;**171**:16077

[84] Sato S, Hanibuchi M, Fukuya A, et al. Idiopathic pleuroparenchymal fibroelastosis is characterized by an elevated serum level of surfactant protein-D, but not Krebs von den Lungen-6. Lung. 2014;**192**:711-717

[85] Kusagaya H, Nakamura Y, Kone M, et al. Idiopathic pleuroparenchymal fibroelastosis: Consideration of a clinicopatholgical entity in a series of Japanese patients. BMC Pulmonary Medicine. 2012;**12**:72-78. On line pub: 1701248

[86] Walter J, Fan L, Bag R, et al. Serum KL-6 as a marker for bronchiolitis obliterans syndrome after lung transplantation. Transplantation. 2006;**82**:709-711

[87] Ohshimo S, Bonella F, Sommerwerck U, et al. Comparison of serum KL-6 versus bronchoalvoelar lavage neutrophilia for the diagnosis of bronchiolitis obliterans in lung transplantation. The Journal of Heart and Lung Transplantation. 2011;**30**:1374-1380

[88] Beeh KM, Beier J, Kornmann O, et al. Sputum levels of metalloproteinase-9 and tissue inhibitor of metalloproteinase-1, and their ratio correlate with airway obstruction in lung transplant recipients: Relation to tumor necrosis factor-alpha and interleukin 10. The Journal of Heart and Lung Transplantation. 2001;**20**:144-151

[89] Hubner RH, Mefffert S, Mundt U, et al. Matrix metalloproteinase-9 in bronchiolitis obliterans syndrome after lung transplantation. The European Respiratory Journal. 2005;**25**:494-501

[90] Nakamura Y, Mori K, Enomoto Y, et al. Prognostic and clinical value of cluster analysis in idiopathic pleuroparenchymal fibroelastosis phenotypes. Journal of Clinical Medicine. 2021;**10**:1498-1506

[91] Nasser M, Si-Mohaned S, Turquier S, et al. Nintedanib in idiopathic and secondary pleuroparenchymal fibroelastosis. Orphanet Journal of Rare Diseases. 2021;**16**:419-a427

[92] Isenring B, Robinson C, Buergi U, et al. Lung transplant recipients on long-term extracorporeal photophoresis. Clinical Transplantation. 2017:e13041. DOI: 10.1111/ctr.13041

[93] Hachem R, Corris P. Extracorporeal photophoresis for bronchiolitis obliterans syndrome after lung transplantation. Transplantation. 2018;**102**:1059-1065

[94] Sato S, Hanibuchi M, Takashi M, et al. A patient with idiopathic pleuroparenchymal fibroelastosis showing a sustained pulmonary function due to treatment with pirfenidone. Internal Medicine. 2016;**55**:497-501

[95] Pluchart H, Chanoine S, Briault A, et al. Restrictive allograft dysfunction after lung transplantation: Is there a place for nintedanib? – A case report. Fundamentals & Clinical pharmacology. 2020;**34**:408-411

[96] Ali M, Ramalingam V, Haasler G, et al. Pleuroparenchymal fibroelastosis (PPFE) treated with lung transplantation and review of the literature. BMJ Case Reports. 2019;**12**:e229402

[97] Shiiya H, Sato M. Lung transplantation for pleuroparenchymal fibroelastosis. Journal of Clinical Medicine. 2021;**10**:957-964

[98] Faccioli E, Verzeletti V, Giraudo C, et al. Lung transplantation for pleuroparenchymal fibroelastosis: A single-center experience with revision of the literature. Biomedicine. 2023;**11**:1505-1514

[99] Shioya M, Otsuka M, Yamada G, et al. Poorer prognosis of idiopathic pleuroparenchymal fibroelastosis compared with idiopathic pulmonary fibrosis in advanced stage. Canadian Respiratory Journal. 2018;**60**(4):543-550

[100] Kato M, Sasaki S, Kurokawa K, et al. Usual interstitial pneumonia pattern in the lower lobes as a prognostic factor in idiopathic pleuroparenchymal fibroelastosis. Respiration. 2019;**97**(4):319-332